Hypertension: Pre-Hypertension to Heart Failure

Editors

KENNETH A. JAMERSON
JAMES BRIAN BYRD

CARDIOLOGY CLINICS

www.cardiology.theclinics.com

Consulting Editors
JORDAN M. PRUTKIN
DAVID M. SHAVELLE
TERRENCE D. WELCH
AUDREY H. WU

May 2017 • Volume 35 • Number 2

ELSEVIER

1600 John F. Kennedy Boulevard • Suite 1800 • Philadelphia, Pennsylvania, 19103-2899

http://www.theclinics.com

CARDIOLOGY CLINICS Volume 35, Number 2
May 2017 ISSN 0733-8651, ISBN-13: 978-0-323-49645-2

Editor: Stacy Eastman
Developmental Editor: Alison Swety

Cardiology Clinics (ISSN 0733-8651) is published quarterly by Elsevier Inc., 360 Park Avenue South, New York, NY 10010-1710. Months of issue are February, May, August, and November. Business and Editorial Offices: 1600 John F. Kennedy Blvd., Ste. 1800, Philadelphia, PA 19103-2899. Customer Service Office: 3251 Riverport Lane, Maryland Heights, MO 63043. Periodicals postage paid at New York, NY and additional mailing offices. Subscription prices are $326.00 per year for US individuals, $604.00 per year for US institutions, $100.00 per year for US students and residents, $398.00 per year for Canadian individuals, $758.00 per year for Canadian institutions, $464.00 per year for international individuals, $758.00 per year for international institutions and $220.00 per year for Canadian and international students/residents. To receive student/resident rate, orders must be accompanied by name of affiliated institution, data of term, and the *signature* of program/residency coordinator on institution letterhead. Orders will be billed at individual rate until proof of status is received. Foreign air speed delivery is included in all *Clinics* subscription prices. All prices are subject to change without notice. **POSTMASTER:** Send address changes to *Cardiology Clinics*, Elsevier Health Sciences Division, Subscription Customer Service, 3251 Riverport Lane, Maryland Heights, MO 63043. **Customer Service: 1-800-654-2452 (U.S. and Canada); 314-447-8871 (outside U.S. and Canada). Fax: 314-447-8029. E-mail: journalscustomerservice-usa@ elsevier.com (for print support); journalsonlinesupport-usa@elsevier.com (for online support).**

Reprints. For copies of 100 or more, of articles in this publication, please contact the Commercial Reprints Department, Elsevier Inc., 360 Park Avenue South, New York, NY 10010-1710. Tel.: 212-633-3874; Fax: 212-633-3820; E-mail: reprints@elsevier.com.

Cardiology Clinics is also published in Spanish by McGraw-Hill Interamericana Editores S. A., P.O. Box 5-237, 06500, Mexico D. F., Mexico; in Portuguese by Reichmann and Alfonso Editores Rio de Janeiro, Brazil; and in Greek by Dimitrios P. Lagos, 8 Pondon Street, GR115-28 Ilissia, Greece.

Cardiology Clinics is covered in *MEDLINE/PubMed (Index Medicus), Excerpta Medica, The Cumulative Index to Nursing and Allied Health Literature* (CINAHL).

Contributors

AUTHORS

WILLIAM T. ABRAHAM, MD, FACP, FACC, FAHA, FESC, FRCP
Professor of Internal Medicine, Physiology, and Cell Biology, Chair of Excellence in Cardiovascular Medicine, Director, Division of Cardiovascular Medicine, The Ohio State University, Columbus, Ohio

MICHELLE A. ALBERT, MD, MPH
Division of Cardiology, Department of Medicine, Center for the Study of Adversity and Cardiovascular Disease [NURTURE Center], University of California, San Francisco, San Francisco, California

LAWRENCE J. APPEL, MD, MPH
C. David Molina Professor of Medicine, Director, Welch Center for Prevention, Epidemiology, and Clinical Research, Johns Hopkins University, Baltimore, Maryland

IVOR J. BENJAMIN, MD, FAHA, FACC
Director, Cardiovascular Center, Department of Medicine; Division of Cardiology, Medical College of Wisconsin, Milwaukee, Wisconsin

PRASHANT D. BHAVE, MD, FHRS
Clinical Assistant Professor of Medicine, Division of Cardiovascular Medicine, Department of Internal Medicine, University of Iowa Hospitals and Clinics, Iowa City, Iowa

JOHN D. BISOGNANO, MD, PhD
Cardiovascular Medicine, Strong Memorial Hospital, University of Rochester, Rochester, New York

ROBERT D. BROOK, MD
Professor of Medicine, Division of
Cardiovascular Medicine, University of
Michigan, Ann Arbor, Michigan

ADOLFO G. CUEVAS, PhD
Cancer Prevention Postdoctoral Fellow,
Department of Social and Behavioral Sciences,
Harvard T.H. Chan School of Public Health,
Landmark Center, Boston, Massachusetts

SHERIFF N. DODOO, MD
Department of Internal Medicine, Meharry
Medical College, Nashville, Tennessee

KEITH C. FERDINAND, MD, FACC, FAHA
Professor of Medicine, Tulane Heart and
Vascular Institute, Tulane University School of
Medicine, New Orleans, Louisiana

**MICHAEL C. GIUDICI, MD, FACC, FACP,
FHRS**
Clinical Professor of Medicine and Director of
Arrhythmia Services, Division of
Cardiovascular Medicine, Department of
Internal Medicine, University of Iowa Hospitals
and Clinics, Iowa City, Iowa

SWAPNIL HIREMATH, MD, MPH
Assistant Professor, Division of Nephrology,
The Ottawa Hospital and University of Ottawa,
Ottawa, Ontario, Canada

SARAH E. KUCHARSKI, MA
Coordinator, E-Patient Programs, Medicinex,
Stanford University, Stanford, California;
Chairman/CEO, Founder, FMDCHAT, Canton,
North Carolina

SUMEET S. MITTER, MD, MSc
Fellow in Advanced Heart Failure and
Transplant Cardiology, Division of Cardiology,
Department of Medicine, Northwestern
University Feinberg School of Medicine,
Chicago, Illinois

SAMAR A. NASSER, PhD, MPH, PA-C
Director, Clinical Health Sciences,
Department of Clinical Research and
Leadership, School of Medicine and Health
Sciences, The George Washington University,
Washington, DC

RAMON A. PARTIDA, MD
Clinical and Research Fellow, Division of
Cardiology, Department of Medicine,
Massachusetts General Hospital, Boston,
Massachusetts; Post-doctoral Research
Fellow, Institute for Medical Engineering and
Science, Massachusetts Institute of
Technology, Cambridge, Massachusetts;
Harvard Medical School, Boston,
Massachusetts

MARCEL RUZICKA, MD, PhD
Associate Professor, Division of Nephrology,
The Ottawa Hospital, University of Ottawa,
Ottawa, Ontario, Canada

SINAN S. TANKUT, MD
Department of Medicine, Strong Memorial
Hospital, University of Rochester, Rochester,
New York

DAVID R. WILLIAMS, PhD, MPH
Florence Sprague Norman and Laura Smart
Norman Professor of Public Health,
Department of Social and Behavioral Sciences,
Harvard T.H. Chan School of Public Health,
Boston, Massachusetts; Department of African
and African American Studies, Harvard
University, Cambridge, Massachusetts

CLYDE W. YANCY, MD, MSc
Division of Cardiology, Professor, Department
of Medicine, Northwestern University Feinberg
School of Medicine, Chicago, Illinois

ROBERT W. YEH, MD, MSc, MBA
Director, Department of Medicine, Smith
Center for Outcomes Research in Cardiology,
CardioVascular Institute, Beth Israel Medical
Center; Medical Director of Trial Design,
Harvard Clinical Research Institute, Harvard
Medical School, Boston, Massachusetts

AYHAN YORUK, MD, MPH
Department of Medicine, Strong Memorial
Hospital, University of Rochester, Rochester,
New York

Contents

> Genomic insights and analyses of Mendelian hypertension (HTN) syndromes and Genome-Wide Association study (GWAS) on essential hypertension have contributed to the depth of understanding of the genetics origins of hypertension. Mendelian syndromes are important for the field, since such knowledge leads to specific insights about disease pathogenesis and the potential for precision medicine. The clinical impact of findings of GWAS on essential hypertension is continuously evolving, and the insights accrued will refine efforts to combat the societal impact of hypertension. Comprehensive identification of all genomic variants of hypertension, along with their individual associated mechanisms, is paving the way forward in the era of personalized medicine. The overriding challenge for care providers is to reduce health inequities through improved compliance and, perhaps, new paradigms for implementation science that incorporate genomic medicine.

> Evidence supports that multiple dietary factors affect blood pressure (BP). Dietary changes that effectively lower BP are weight loss, reduced sodium intake, increased potassium intake, moderation of alcohol intake, and Dietary Approaches to Stop Hypertension–style and vegetarian dietary patterns. In view of the increasing levels of BP in children and adults and the continuing epidemic of BP-related cardiovascular and renal diseases, efforts to reduce BP in both nonhypertensive and hypertensive individuals are warranted. The challenge to health care providers, researchers, government officials, and the general public is developing and implementing clinical and public health strategies that lead to sustained dietary changes.

> A host of environmental factors can significantly increase arterial blood pressure (BP) including cold temperature, high altitude, loud noises, and ambient air pollutants. Although brief exposures acutely elevate BP, over the long term, chronic exposures may be capable of promoting the development of sustained hypertension. Given their omnipresent nature, environmental factors may play a role in worsening BP control and heightening overall cardiovascular risk at the global public health level.

> Black people have the highest prevalence of hypertension in the United States. Evidence suggests that psychosocial factors increase the risks for hypertension

and help to account for racial differences in this condition. This article reviews research on psychosocial factors and hypertension, and contextualizes the findings within a health disparities framework. A wide range of psychosocial factors contribute to hypertension but understanding remains limited about how these factors relate to each other and accumulate to contribute to hypertension disparities. Future research on psychosocial factors and hypertension needs to enhance the effectiveness of interventions to reduce hypertension risk in ethnic minority communities.

The treatment of essential hypertension is one of the most critical interventions to decrease cardiovascular morbidity and mortality. The prevalence of hypertension in the US varies across race/ethnicity with African Americans having the highest prevalence and overall less control among racial/ethnic minorities compared with non-Hispanic whites. Therapeutic lifestyle modifications are the bedrock of essential hypertension control, but most patients with hypertension will require pharmacotherapy, usually with multiple medications often in combination. Overall, the principal drug classes recommended as initial pharmacotherapy are thiazide-type diuretics, calcium channel blockers, and angiotensin-converting enzyme inhibitors or angiotensin receptor blockers.

Knowledge about fibromuscular dysplasia (FMD) has broadened over the last several decades. It is no longer considered a rare and benign entity limited to renal arteries and causing just hypertension. It affects other parts of the arterial tree nearly as frequently as the renal arteries. Complications of undiagnosed and untreated extrarenal FMD can be debilitating and life threatening. However, this disease, specifically extrarenal FMD, is not well known to many physicians and patients. Combined with the nonspecific symptoms and signs of the disease, this leads to delayed diagnosis and missed opportunity to prevent serious vascular complications.

Hypertension remains a significant risk factor for an array of diseases despite advancements in pharmacotherapy. Patients with resistant hypertension who do not respond to conventional medical treatments and lifestyle modifications are especially at risk for poor health outcomes. With the increasing awareness of resistant hypertension, ever-evolving research efforts continue to focus on innovative interventions, including renal denervation, median nerve stimulation, and baroreceptor activation therapy. This article reviews the current evidence and summarizes previous clinical trials for each of these interventions.

Incident heart failure and the burden of hospitalization may be demonstrating a decline. However, as the population ages, the prevalence of heart failure continues to increase. Mortality among heart failure patients is increasingly due to non-cardiovascular causes. Current evidence-based therapy for heart failure has improved heart failure related mortality. Current efforts should be directed toward optimizing evidence based medical and device therapy, reducing morbidity, and increasing quality of life with heart failure. Future clinical trials should focus on therapies for heart failure with preserved ejection fraction, regenerative therapy for heart failure, and optimizing durable mechanical support for end-stage heart failure.

Special Articles

Heart failure is associated with high rates of hospitalization and rehospitalization, resulting in substantial clinical and economic burden. Current approaches to monitoring patients with heart failure have done little to reduce these high rates of heart failure hospitalization. Implantable hemodynamic monitors have been developed to remotely provide direct measurement of intracardiac and pulmonary artery pressures in ambulatory patients with heart failure. These devices have the potential to direct day-to-day management of patients with heart failure to reduce hospitalization rates. The use of a pulmonary artery pressure measurement system has been shown to reduce the risk of heart failure hospitalization in patients with systolic and diastolic heart failure.

First-generation drug-eluting stents significantly improved treatment of coronary disease, decreasing rates of revascularization. This was offset by high rates of late adverse events, driven primarily by stent thrombosis. Research and design improvements of individual DES platform components led to next-generation devices with superior clinical safety and efficacy profiles compared with bare-metal stents and first-generation drug-eluting stents. These design improvements and features are explored, and their resulting clinical safety and efficacy reviewed, focusing on platforms approved by the Food and Drug Administration currently widely used in the United States.

The relationship of stroke and atrial fibrillation seems to become more complex as we gain more knowledge of the issue. Recent studies have questioned the temporal relationship between the two, which also questions causation. Left atrial appendage closure is an attractive, but unproven technology when compared with the 50-year experience with warfarin. In a patient who is on warfarin and having no issues with bleeding, medication intolerance, or lack of efficacy, it is difficult to justify stopping the drug and placing a closure device as sole therapy to prevent a stroke.

CARDIOLOGY CLINICS

THE CLINICS ARE AVAILABLE ONLINE!
Access your subscription at:
www.theclinics.com

Preface

Hypertension: From Pre-Hypertension to Heart Failure

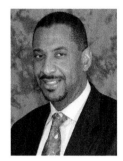 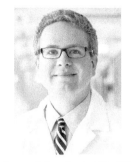

Kenneth A. Jamerson, MD   James Brian Byrd, MD, MS
Editors

Elevated blood pressure is a major risk factor for coronary heart disease and stroke (the overwhelming leading cause of death worldwide for the past decade). Elevated blood pressure is estimated to cause 7.5 million deaths annually, or about 12.8% of the total of all deaths worldwide. Blood pressure levels are positively and continuously related to the risk for stroke and coronary heart disease. Thus, the prevention and treatment of hypertension are of paramount importance to a global health agenda. In this issue of *Cardiology Clinics*, we invited experts with vast research experience to codify and present a contemporary topic on elevated blood pressure. The scope of the issue includes elevated blood pressure and its genetic, environmental, and psycho/social mediators. We also provide a comprehensive approach to the treatment of essential hypertension and contemporary topics in secondary hypertension. Finally, those with hypertension are classified as stage A heart failure, representing high risk, and antihypertensive medication is the primary treatment for heart failure until the most advanced stages. Therefore, this issue includes a comprehensive article on the clinical management of heart failure. This issue is unique, providing readers granular information on specific genes, environmental particles, stress, foods, and drugs as therapeutic approaches to hypertension, while it also provides a broad overview of the spectrum of prehypertension to heart failure and its global burden. The topics selected for this issue have a history of causing some controversy or confusion: the role of dietary sodium in hypertension, the clinical significance of genetics in cardiovascular disease, and the role of renal artery stenosis as a modifiable factor in secondary hypertension, for example. The invited authors have made a tremendous effort to make these potentially confusing topics clear and accessible.

The guest editors express a sincere debt of gratitude to the authoritative authors (invited authors have more than two decades of original contributions to their area of expertise) for accepting the challenge of creating each cutting-edge article. This issue of *Cardiology Clinics* has both a goal and a message. Our goal was to create a comprehensive compendium for clinical management of prehypertension and heart failure. Our message: hypertension is a global disease burden disproportionately afflicting people with inadequate resources. The prescription will require more than inexpensive drugs. We call attention to the heart

Cardiol Clin 35 (2017) ix–x
http://dx.doi.org/10.1016/j.ccl.2017.02.001

cardiology.theclinics.com

and mind of people, the air that they breathe, and the food they ingest.

Kenneth A. Jamerson, MD
University of Michigan Health System
Division of Cardiovascular Medicine
1500 East Medical Center Drive
2272G Frankel Cardiovascular Center
Ann Arbor, MI 48109-5853, USA

James Brian Byrd, MD, MS
University of Michigan Health System
Division of Cardiovascular Medicine
1150 West Medical Center Drive
5570C Medical Science Research Building II
Ann Arbor, MI 48109, USA

E-mail addresses:
jamerson@umich.edu (K.A. Jamerson)
jbbyrd@umich.edu (J.B. Byrd)

Genomic Approaches to Hypertension

Sheriff N. Dodoo, MD[a], Ivor J. Benjamin, MD[b,c],*

KEYWORDS

- Hypertension • Blood pressure • Genomic approaches

KEY POINTS

- Genomic insights and analyses of Mendelian hypertension (HTN) syndromes and Genome-Wide Association study (GWAS) on essential HTN have contributed to the depth of understanding of the genetics origins of hypertension.
- Mendelian syndromes are important for the field, since such knowledge leads to specific insights about disease pathogenesis and the potential for precision medicine.
- The clinical impact of findings of GWAS on essential HTN is continuously evolving, and the accrued insights will refine efforts to combat the societal impact of hypertension.
- Comprehensive identification of all genomic variants of hypertension, along with their individual associated mechanisms, is paving the way forward in the era of personalized medicine.
- The overriding challenge for care providers is to reduce health inequities through improved compliance and, perhaps, new paradigms for implementation science that incorporates genomic medicine.

INTRODUCTION

Hypertension is the leading cause of cardiovascular morbidity and mortality worldwide,[1–3] affecting more than a third of the US adult population[4,5] with a disproportionate burden in underrepresented and ethnic minorities including African Americans.[6] In both personal and societal terms, blood pressure control has emerged as an important health indicator in the US population and for 1 billion people worldwide. To attain the American Heart Association Strategy Impact Goals to improve cardiovascular health of all Americans by 2020 and beyond, an ideal blood pressure target (<120/80 mm Hg) ranks among the 7 ideal health indicators[7] being directly targeted in populations. Although an in-depth review of the clinical manifestations, diagnostic evaluation, and treatment options of asymptomatic and symptomatic hypertension are covered elsewhere, this article reviews the genetic causes and provides a conceptual framework by which genomic analyses have propelled novel insights into the mechanisms of systemic and arterial hypertension.

Hypertension remains a significant public health problem with far-reaching impact on disease burden globally from stroke, heart failure, aortic dissection, atrial fibrillation, myocardial infarction, and end-stage kidney disease. In fact, a recent publication by Lawes and colleagues[8] concluded that 13.5% of premature deaths, 54% of strokes and 47% of ischemic heart disease worldwide are attributable to uncontrolled hypertension. Among the most easily recognizable and reversible risk factors, these authors further concluded that about 80% of the attributable burden

Disclosure statement: The authors have no financial or commercial conflicts of interest to declare.
[a] Department of Internal Medicine, Meharry Medical College, 1005 Dr DB Todd Jr Boulevard, Nashville, TN 37208, USA; [b] Cardiovascular Center, Department of Medicine, Medical College of Wisconsin, 8701 Watertown Plank Road, Milwaukee, WI 53226, USA; [c] Division of Cardiology, Department of Medicine, Medical College of Wisconsin, 8701 Watertown Plank Road, Milwaukee, WI 53226, USA
* Corresponding author. Cardiovascular Center, Medical College of Wisconsin, 8701 Watertown Plank Road, Milwaukee, WI 53226.
E-mail address: ibenjamin@mcw.edu

occurred in low-income and middle-income economies. In spite of evidence of medical therapeutics and access to advanced systems of medical care, fewer than 50% of Americans treated for hypertension reach the target blood pressure goals. To achieve effective gains, both highly motivated and educated individuals affected with hypertension along with knowledgeable medical providers are prerequisites for proper blood pressure control and management.

Although the etiology of essential hypertension is unknown, both genetic and environmental factors play important roles in the pathophysiologic mechanisms in modern societies.[9] In epidemiologic studies among members of the Luo tribe in Kenya, for example, Poulter and colleagues[10] have highlighted lower blood pressure in their traditional rural environment compared with the urban center of Nairobi where urinary sodium and potassium concentrations was higher and lower, respectively. Because the renin-angiotensin- aldosterone system (RAS) has features for adaptation in sodium conservation, it has been hypothesized that a sodium-deprived environment favors sodium conservation as the default phenotype, underscoring the importance of salt reabsorption in the pathogenesis of hypertension in societies with high dietary salt intake.[11] In recent decades, substantial progress has been made to elucidate the mechanisms underlying the physiologic pathways and molecular targets of genes causally linked to rare Mendelian forms of hypertension in people.

GENOMIC VARIATION AND HUMAN INHERITABLE DISEASES

Thanks to the Human Genome Project, the promise to identify the consequence of germ line mutations (ie, single-nucleotide variants [SNV] and copy-number variants [CNV]) has yielded almost 3000 protein-coding genes linked to disease-associated mutations in people.[12] Innovations of genome sequencing coupled with technologies that dramatically reduce the amount of DNA required for coverage of coding regions have revolutionized the identification of rare variants and disease-causing mutations. Genomic approaches such as whole exome capture and sequencing technologies for increased sensitivity and specificity have provided an important means to investigate inheritability factors of hypertension. Indeed, proof of concept for whole-exome sequencing has been validated as a clinical diagnostic tool for the evaluation of patients with previously undiagnosed genetic disease.[13]

For Mendelian diseases, the discovery of the genetic basis is central to establishing causality between genotype and phenotype and the foundation for genetic screening and diagnosis in affected populations. Studies from family and twin research suggest that blood pressure is moderately heritable (30%–50%).[14] However, the extent to which the percentage of inheritability influences the development of hypertension has been previously challenged.[15] When single-gene mutations result in the large effects on the phenotype, then applications of next-generation sequencing have identified rare variants with moderate-to-large effects, especially in populations of phenotypic extremes.

Along with traditional cardiovascular risks factors, 2 broad groups of genomic variants have been proposed to influence the development of hypertension. These are the effects of genomic variants on the development of rare familial syndromes that lead to monogenic hypertension (HTN) and the genetic variants underlying common essential HTN. These rare familial genome variants with monogenic hypertension have large effects, potentially triggering hypertensive crises with severe cardiovascular morbidity and mortality. However, the many genetic variants with small effects likely underlie the polygenic trait of common essential HTN in people. Thus, familial hypertensive syndromes are rarely caused by monogenetic variants that significantly influence an increase in blood pressure with variable effect size. In these hypertensive syndromes, patients develop HTN at an early age (**Table 1**) and have effect sizes as much as 10 mm Hg in systolic blood pressure.

THE GENOMIC VARIANTS IN BLOOD PRESSURE REGULATION CAUSING RARE FAMILIAL HYPERTENSIVE SYNDROMES

Because large fractions of interindividual variability can be attributed to genetic determinants, the pursuit of rare disease-causing mutations using genetic approaches has successfully yielded substantial insights into the pathophysiology of hypertension while simultaneously affording new opportunities for tailored therapies in the era of precision medicine. Several monogenic variants have established Mendelian modes of inheritance.[33,34] Twelve genes have been identified, modulating and influencing the development of 8 distinct rare familial hypertensive syndromes, all of which are inherited in a Mendelian fashion. **Table 1** summarizes these genetic variants including key features of each clinical syndrome. Recently, 2 of the 4 genes known to cause Gordon syndrome were identified.[22,24] Other Mendelian HTN syndromes have been mapped to genomic regions,

Table 1
Genes associated with monogenic hypertension

Gene(s)	Chr	Disease Name	Key Features of Clinical Syndrome	Mode of Inheritance and Genetic Mechanism	% HTN (N)—% Early Onset HTN (N)c	Estimated Frequency; Occurrence in the General Population
CYP11B1 (11-beta hydroxylase gene)[16]	8q	(MIM: 202010) CAH type IV (congenital adrenal hyperplasia, caused by 11-beta-hydroxylase deficiency)	HTN, hypokalemia, virilization (variable); 2 of 3 patients have severe, classic form with HTN in the first years of life; otherwise HTN is usually mild to moderate in intensity; accounts for 5%–8% of all CAH cases	AR; LOF	63% (38)—NA[17]	~1/100,000 births ~1/5–7000 in Jewish families of North African origin (Morocco, Tunisia)
CYP11B2 (aldosterone synthase gene)[18]	8p	(MIM: 103900) Glucocorticoid remediable aldosteronism: familial hyperaldosteronism type I: glucocorticoid suppressible hyperaldosteronism	HTN, low plasma renin, increased aldosterone, response to dexamethasone; high genetic heterogeneity and potassium level often normal; high prevalence of intracranial aneurysms	AD; GOF gene expressed under ACTH control (fusion of the promoter region of the gene for CYP11B1 and the coding sequences of CYP11B2)	88% (8)–41% (12)[19]	Rare defect

(continued on next page)

Table 1
(continued)

Gene(s)	Chr	Disease Name	Key Features of Clinical Syndrome	Mode of Inheritance and Genetic Mechanism	% HTN (N)—% Early Onset HTN (N)c	Estimated Frequency; Occurrence in the General Population
WNK1, WNK4 (lysine-deficient protein kinase 1 and 4 genes)[20]	12p	Pseudohypoaldosteronism type 2 (PHA2): Gordon syndrome WNK1: PHA2C (MIM: 614492) WNK4: PHA2B (MIM: 614491) KLHL3: PHA2D (MIM: 614495) CUL3: PHA2E (MIM: 614496)	HTN, hyperkalemia, response to thiazides	WNK1: AR; GOF WNK4: AR; LOF; ↑ expression of the thiazide-sensitive Na-Cl co-transporter SLC12A3 (NCCT) KLHL3: AD or AR; LOF (inhibition of KLHL3 increases the activity of SLC12A3) CUL3: AD; LOF	WNK1: 84% (12)–13%[21,22] WNK4: 50% (18)–10%[22,23] KLHL3 dominant: 27% (15)–17%[24] KLHL3 recessive: 100% (5)–14%[24] CUL3: NA—94%[22]	Rare defect
KLHL3 (kelch-like 3 gene)[22,24]	5q					
CUL3 (cullin 3 gene)[22]	2q					
SCNN1B, SCNN1G (amiloride-sensitive sodium channel, beta and gamma subunit gene encoding 2 subunits of the ENaC sodium channel)[25,26]	16p	(MIM: 177200) Liddle's syndrome: pseudoaldosteronism[27,28]	HTN, hypokalemia, metabolic alkalosis, low plasma renin, low aldosterone, respond to amiloride	AD; GOF	SCNN1B: 100% (18)[27] SCNN1G: 100% (6)–50% (6)[26]	Rare defect

Gene	Location	Disease (MIM)	Phenotype	Inheritance; mechanism	Percentage	Comments
CYP17A1- (steroid 17-hydroxylase/17,20 lyase gene)[29]	10q	(MIM: 202110) Congenital adrenal hyperplasia, caused by 17-alpha-hydroxylase deficiency: CAH type V	HTN, hypokalemia, hypogonadism/androgen deficiency	AR; LOF	NA[30]	Very rare defect
HSD11B2(11-beta-hydroxy steroid dehydrogenase 2 gene)[31]	16q	(MIM: 218030) Cortisol 11-beta-ketoreductase deficiency; syndrome of apparent mineralocorticoid excess	HTN, hypokalemia, low plasma renin, responsiveness to spironolactone; severe HTN	AR; LOF	100% (9) to >89% (9)[31]	Very rare defect
NR3C2 (mineralocorticoid receptor gene)[51]	4q	(MIM: 605115) Early-onset autosomal dominant HTN with exacerbation in pregnancy	HTN, severe HTN in pregnancy	AD; GOF	100%(8)–100% (8)d[51]	One large pedigree reported
KCNJ5 (potassium inwardly rectifying channel gene, subfamily J, member 5)[32]	11q	(MIM: 613677) Familial hyperaldosteronism type III	HTN, hypokalemia, high aldosterone, high 18-oxocortisol and 18-hydroxycortisol	AD; LOF	100% (3)–100% (3)[32]	One pedigree reported

The percentage of patients with HTN and with early-onset HTN (≤18 years of age) is indicated in this review.
The age limit for early-onset HTN was less than 20 years.
Abbreviations: AD, autosomal dominant; AR, autosomal recessive; GOF, gain of function; LOF, loss of function; NA, not available.
From Ehret GB, Caulfield MJ. Genes for blood pressure: an opportunity to understand hypertension. Eur Heart J 2013;34(13):953–4; with permission.

although their specific defects are yet to be demonstrated. These conditions remain an active area of exploration and intense research.

KEY FEATURES OF MONOGENIC HYPERTENSION

The monogenic hypertension genes that follow the rules of classical Mendelian may be inherited as autosomal-dominant and recessive disorders. An autosomal-dominant pattern of inheritance refers to an affected individual who has 1 copy of a mutant gene and 1 normal gene on a pair of autosomal chromosomes. An autosomal-recessive pattern of inheritance has both copies of the mutant gene on a pair of autosomal chromosomes. A polygenic trait is one whose phenotype is influenced by more than 1 gene. Complex traits such as hypertension are polygenic and display a continuous distribution, such as height or skin color. Phenotypic features of renal salt homeostasis, electrolyte, and hormonal disturbance are contributing factors to familial monogenic hypertensive syndromes.[34,35] More precise phenotypic analysis by biochemical analysis is required for measurements of aldosterone, renin, and additional hormones. Furthermore, 7 out of the 12 genes presented as loss-of-function mutations. These syndromes (see **Table 1**) often lead to severe hypertensive crises in one of 2 ways, either a reduction of an inhibitory effect on blood pressure or a positive feedback loop that leads to an increase in blood pressure. The identification of the genetic basis of these hypertensive disease states may be important in our request for therapeutic approaches to these rare disease entities. Such patients with suspected monogenic HTN syndromes should be referred to advanced specialized centers.

MECHANISTIC PATHWAYS OF THE MONOGENIC HYPERTENSIVE SYNDROMES

Mutations linked to genes affecting mineralocorticoid metabolism have provided the earliest evidence for genetic determinants of hypertension in people. Recent efforts have now well-established 12 genes covering 2 general pathways in the pathogenesis of monogenic hypertension: namely, renal sodium homeostasis and steroid hormone metabolism linked to mineralocorticoid receptor activity as illustrated in **Fig. 1**.

The epithelial sodium channel ($E_{NA}C$) functions in the final common pathway for sodium reabsorption in the distal nephron. The gain-of-function mutation of $E_{NA}C$ results in the salt-dependent hypertension or Liddle Syndrome. Pseudohypoaldosteronism Type II (PHAII) is a rare Mendelian syndrome

characterized by hypertension, metabolic acidosis, and hyperkalemia, and it is caused by mutations encoding the *Klech-like 3* and *Cullen 3* genes (16). The renal physiology has features underscored by salt reabsorption and both K^+ and H^+ excretion. Maximum salt reabsorption appears to be orchestrated due to elevated aldosterone by increased levels of angiotensin II (16). In certain instances, hypertension contributes to inheritable forms of the metabolic syndrome when clustered with comorbidities and risk factors of early onset coronary artery disease, central obesity, and diabetes.[36]

Other known monogenic defects include Peroxisome-proliferator-activated-receptor (PPAR) gamma mutations in the pathogenesis of diabetes and HTN21 or RET gene mutations underlying the manifestation of pheochromocytoma, HTN, and other malignancies. The finding that genetic defects in HTN syndromes localize to proteins of the kidney and to steroid hormone activity suggested that similar mechanisms also contribute to the genetic origin of essential HTN. Of note, there is also the partial overlap between the pathways of monogenic HTN and commonly used antihypertensive drugs used to treat essential HTN (eg, thiazide diuretics, aldosterone receptor antagonists).

GENOME-WIDE ASSOCIATION STUDIES AND HYPERTENSION

For human genetic studies, linkage analysis has been a valuable tool used to identify genomic loci of high penetrance. The first large-scale attempt to validate HTN variants by GWAS was carried out by the Welcome Trust Case Control Consortium in in a British population, identifying genome-wide significant variants among 7 common diseases using 2000 cases and 3000 controls.[37] Since then, several consortia and individual trials have published 43 variants that could be replicated in independent samples (**Table 2**) using GWAS or similar methods. Most investigations have been carried out using samples of European origin, including CHARGE (Cohorts for Heart and Aging Research in Genomic Epidemiology) consortium, the Global BP Gen (Global BP Genetics) consortium, and the ICBP (International Consortium for BP GWAS). Notable Non-European samples particularly involve cohorts of Asian origin and include studies of the Korea Association Resource consortium and the Asian Genetic Epidemiology Network. The study using participants of African origin is the CARe (Candidate-gene Association Resource) consortium.

To date, the largest contribution to the total number of genomic loci discovered for systolic blood pressure (SBP), diastolic blood pressure (DBP),

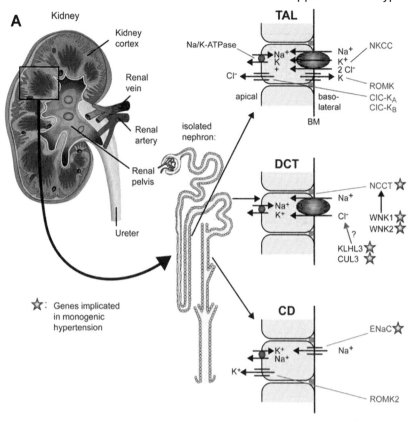

Fig. 1. Disease-causing pathways affected in monogenic hypertension. Genes encoding the mutated gene products are shown to be located in the context of physiologic pathways associated with salt reabsorption homeostasis. Two groups of pathways are affected, pathways affecting the kidney (*A*) and pathways affecting steroid metabolism and the mineralocorticoid receptor (*B*). A selection of important structures (eg, ion channels) or enzymes is labeled in gray. Proteins mutated in monogenic HTN syndromes are marked by a red star. CD, collecting duct; DCT, distal-convoluted tubule; TAL, thick ascending limb of the loop of Henle. (*From* Ehret GB, Caulfield MJ. Genes for blood pressure: an opportunity to understand hypertension. Eur Heart J 2013;34(13):955; with permission.)

Table 2
Summary of genetic variants associated with alterations of blood pressure

Locus Name	Sentinel SNP	chr	Position (hg19)	CA	SBP		DBP		HTN		Ethnicity	Max N
					Beta	P-Value	Beta	P-Value	Beta	P-Value		
CASZ1[38,39]	rs880315	1	10,796,866	C	0.61	5.20×10^9	NA	NA	NA	NA	EU, AS	52,155
MTHFR (3')-NPPB[44]	rs4846049	1	11,850,365	T	NA	NA	−0.34	3.00×10^{10}	NA	NA	EU	84,467
MTHFR (5')-NPPB[40–43]	rs17367504	1	11,862,778	G	−0.90	8.72×10^{22}	−0.55	3.55×10^{19}	−0.10	2.34×10^{10}	EU	125,000
ST7L-CAPZA1[47]	rs17030613	1	113,190,807	C	0.49	8.40×10^8	0.38	1.20×10^8	NA	NA	AS	49,952
MOV1[40]	rs2932538	1	113,216,543	G	0.39	1.17×10^9	0.24	9.88×10^{10}	0.05	2.89×10^7	EU, AS	195,000
AGT[44–46]	rs2004776	1	230,848,702	T	0.42	3.80×10^6	0.32	5.00×10^8	0.08	3.70×10^7	EU, AS	86,588
FIGN_GRB14[47,48]	rs16849225	2	164,906,820	C	0.75	3.50×10^{10}	0.29	2.70×10^5	NA	NA	AS, EU	49,511
SLC4A7[40]	rs13082711	3	27,537,909	T	−0.32	1.51×10^6	−0.24	3.77×10^9	−0.03	3.56×10^4	EU	198,000
ULK4[40,49]	rs3774372	3	41,877,414	T	−0.07	3.95×10^1	−0.37	9.02×10^{14}	−0.02	1.81×10^1	EU	162,000
MAP4[48]	rs319690	3	47,927,484	T	−0.423	4.74×10^8	−0.265	6.88×10^9	NA	NA	EU	93,496
MECOM[40]	rs419076	3	169,100,886	T	0.41	1.78×10^{13}	0.24	2.12×10^{12}	0.03	3.06×10^4	EU	194,000
FGF5[40,41,46,47,52]	rs1458038	4	81,164,723	T	0.71	1.47×10^{23}	0.46	8.46×10^{25}	0.07	1.85×10^7	EU, AS	140,000
SLC39A8[40]	rs13107325	4	103,188,709	T	−0.98	3.27×10^{14}	−0.68	2.28×10^{17}	−0.10	4.89×10^7	EU	151,000
ENPEP[47]	rs6825911	4	111,381,638	C	0.6	7.30×10^8	0.39	9.00×10^9	NA	NA	AS	49,515
GUCY1A3-1B3[40]	rs13139571	4	156,645,513	C	0.32	1.16×10^6	0.26	2.17×10^{10}	0.04	2.49×10^5	EU	185,000
NPR3-C5orf23[40,47]	rs1173771	5	32,815,028	G	0.50	1.79×10^{16}	0.26	9.11×10^{12}	0.06	3.23×10^{10}	EU, AS	159,000
EBF1[40]	rs11953630	5	157,845,402	T	−0.41	3.02×10^{11}	−0.28	3.81×10^{13}	−0.05	1.68×10^7	EU	161,000
HFE[40]	rs1799945	6	26,091,179	G	0.63	7.69×10^{12}	0.46	1.45×10^{15}	0.09	1.76×10^{10}	EU	144,000
BAT2-BAT5[40]	rs805303	6	31,616,366	G	0.38	1.49×10^{11}	0.23	2.98×10^{11}	0.05	1.12×10^{10}	EU	202,000
PIK3CG[48]	rs17477177	7	106,411,858	T	−0.552	5.67×10^{11}	−0.081	1.40×10^1	NA	NA	EU	112,996
NOS3[45,50]	rs3918226	7	150,690,176	T	NA	NA	0.78	2.20×10^9	NA	NA	EU	84,467
BLK-GATA4[38]	rs2898290	8	11,433,909	C	−0.53	3.40×10^9	NA	NA	NA	NA	EU	52,155
CYP11B2[46]	rs1799998	8	143,999,600	T	0.91	1.50×10^5	0.53	1.80×10^5	NA	NA	AS	19,426

Gene	SNP	Chr	Position	CA	Effect 1	P 1	Effect 2	P 2	Effect 3	P 3	Ancestry	N
CACNB2(5')[40]	rs4373814	10	18,419,972	G	−0.37	4.81×10^{11}	−0.22	4.36×10^{10}	−0.05	8.53×10^{8}	EU	188,000
CACNB2(3')[40,49,53]	rs1813353	10	18,707,448	T	0.57	2.56×10^{12}	0.41	2.30×10^{15}	0.08	6.24×10^{10}	EU, AS	102,000
C10orf107[40,43]	rs4590817	10	63,467,553	G	0.65	3.97×10^{12}	0.42	1.29×10^{12}	0.10	9.82×10^{9}	EU	111,000
PLCE1[40]	rs932764	10	95,895,940	G	0.48	7.10×10^{16}	0.18	8.06×10^{7}	0.06	9.35×10^{9}	EU	161,000
CYP17A1-NT5C2[46,47,49,51–54]	rs11191548	10	104,846,178	T	1.10	6.90×10^{26}	0.46	9.44×10^{13}	0.10	1.40×10^{5}	EU, AS	162,000
ADRB1[45]	rs1801253	10	115,805,056	G	−0.57	4.70×10^{10}	−0.36	9.50×10^{10}	−0.06	3.30×10^{4}	EU	86,588
ADM[40]	rs7129220	11	10,350,538	G	−0.62	2.97×10^{12}	−0.30	6.44×10^{8}	−0.04	1.11×10^{3}	EU	183,000
PLEKHA7[40,49,54]	rs381815	11	16,902,268	T	0.57	5.27×10^{11}	0.35	5.34×10^{10}	0.06	3.41×10^{6}	EU, AS	97,000
FLJ32810-TMEM1[40,55]	rs633185	11	100,593,538	G	−0.56	1.21×10^{17}	−0.33	1.95×10^{15}	−0.07	5.41×10^{11}	EU, AS	160,000
ATP2B1[39,40,49,52,54,56,57]	rs17249754	12	90,060,586	G	0.93	1.82×10^{18}	0.52	1.16×10^{14}	0.13	1.13×10^{14}	EU, AS	96,000
SH2B3[40,41,48,58]	rs3184504	12	111,884,608	T	0.60	3.83×10^{18}	0.45	3.59×10^{25}	0.06	2.62×10^{6}	EU, AF	121,000
ALDH2[47]	rs11066280	12	112,817,783	T	1.56	7.90×10^{31}	1.01	1.30×10^{35}	NA	NA	AS	46,957
TBX5-TBX3[40,47,49,58]	rs10850411	12	115,387,796	T	0.35	5.38×10^{8}	0.25	5.43×10^{10}	0.05	5.18×10^{6}	EU, AS	161,000
CYP1A1-ULK3[40,41,49,57,58]	rs1378942	15	75,077,367	C	0.61	5.69×10^{23}	0.42	2.69×10^{26}	0.07	1.04×10^{8}	EU, AS, AF	163,000
FURIN-FES[40]	rs2521501	15	91,437,388	T	0.65	5.20×10^{19}	0.36	1.89×10^{15}	0.06	7.02×10^{7}	EU, AS, AF	127,000
UMOD[59]	rs13333226	16	20,365,654	G	−0.49	2.60×10^{5}	−0.3	1.50×10^{5}	NA	1.50×10^{13}	EU	79,133
GOSR2[40]	rs17608766	17	45,013,271	T	−0.56	1.13×10^{10}	−0.13	1.66×10^{2}	−0.02	7.99×10^{2}	EU	152,000
ZNF652[40,43]	rs12940887	17	47,402,807	T	0.36	1.79×10^{10}	0.27	2.29×10^{14}	0.05	1.20×10^{7}	EU	188,000
JAG1[40]	rs1327235	20	10,969,030	G	0.34	1.87×10^{8}	0.30	1.41×10^{15}	0.03	4.57×10^{4}	EU, AS	158,000
GNAS-EDN3[40]	rs6015450	20	57,751,117	G	0.90	3.87×10^{23}	0.56	5.63×10^{23}	0.11	4.18×10^{14}	EU, AS	159,000

The table includes loci associated with SBP, DBP, HTN that were replicated in independent samples. Only data from unbiased experiments as the GWAS and similar experiments are included, and only single marker analyses were considered. Only SNPs discovered using an additive model were included, and the maximal r2 between 2 pairs of SNPs was set to be 0.3. The locus name is the name of the nearest gene or a composite of the flanking genes if several genes are near.38

Abbreviations: AF, individuals of African-American or African origin; AS, individuals of Asian origin; CA, coded allele; DBP, diastolic blood pressure; EU, individuals of European ancestry; NA, not available; SBP, systolic blood pressure.

From Ehret GB, Caulfield MJ. Genes for blood pressure: an opportunity to understand hypertension. Eur Heart J 2013;34(13):958–9; with permission.

and HTN is by the International Consortium for Blood pressure (ICBP) GWAS,[40] although many other studies have contributed additional variants. The ICBP study included total discovery GWAS data involving 69,395 individuals and further replication genotyping/look-ups in up to 133,661 subjects. The experiment replicated 13 genomic loci discovered in several other overlapping studies[41,49] and demonstrated 29 SNPs with genome-wide significance, all of which have been independently validated to increase the risk of HTN.

PERSPECTIVES FROM THE DISCOVERY OF 43 VARIANTS FOR ESSENTIAL HYPERTENSION BY GWAS

From 3 decades of research on the genetics of essential HTN, what lessons have emerged from variants identified by the GWAS and other similar linkage analyses thus far? The overall BP effect sizes of individual genetic variant are small, typically 1 mm Hg for SBP and 0.5 mm Hg for DBP (see **Table 2** - subset of SNPs). Collectively, all 29 variants tested in 1 experiment account for only 1% to 2% of SBP and DBP variance.[40] One repeatedly tested hypothesis is that only a small subset of all blood pressure-associated SNPs has been identified. Hence the heritability of blood pressure is about 25 times larger than the difference currently explained by SNPs identified through GWAS. In addition, only a portion of the total heritability of hypertension can currently be explained by the GWAS contributing to the term missing heritability.[60] The expectation is that many more loci yet to be discovered will include variants in the rare allele spectrum with larger effect sizes. For SNPs with effect sizes similar to those in **Table 2** the total number of variants denoting blood pressure variation has been extrapolated to be about 116.[40] In 1 well-designed experiment, a risk score of the combined effects of the 29 SNPs has been clearly associated with blood pressure and HTN in multiple populations.[40] This partially explains the overall phenotypic variance of HTN and hence may not be useful in HTN risk prediction. Of the 43 variants significantly associated with SBP, DBP, and HTN outlined in **Table 2**, only a few are near a gene that has been established to be related to blood pressure. The remaining variants are localized in genomic loci that were previously thought not to be associated with blood pressure. It is hoped that other GWAS consortia could identify over-represented biological pathways in analyses using GWAS SNPs,[61] but efforts in this direction have not been successful for blood pressure thus far. Confounding factors may be attributed to the intrinsic properties of the phenotype or to the small number of variants identified so far. Many variants identified may not be peculiar to individuals of European decent, but also found in cohorts of Asian and African origin. This evidence suggests that, although, genomic analysis in multiple ethnicities is far from complete, many of these variants identified may have significant impact across ethnicities. Such hypotheses are clearly the focus of further studies.

SUMMARY

Genomic insights and analyses of Mendelian HTN syndromes and GWAS on essential HTN have contributed to the depth of current understanding of the genetics origins of hypertension. These rare monogenic hypertensive syndromes are likely to be encountered by practitioners at specialized centers, and warrant attention to the heterogeneous category of essential hypertension encountered on a regular basis.

Mendelian syndromes are important for the field, since such knowledge leads to specific insights about disease pathogenesis and the potential for precision medicine. Furthermore, the clinical impact of findings of GWAS on essential HTN is continuously evolving, and the accrued insights accrued will refine efforts to combat the societal impact of hypertension. Comprehensive identification of all genomic variants of hypertension, along with their individual associated mechanisms, is paving the way forward in the era of personalized medicine. Notwithstanding, the overriding challenge for care providers is to reduce health inequities through improved compliance and, perhaps, new paradigms for implementation science incorporating genomic medicine.

ACKNOWLEDGMENTS

The authors thank Abigail Stein for her editorial assistance. An NIH Director's Pioneer Award Grant HL17650 and the Advancing a Healthier Wisconsin Endowment at the Medical College of Wisconsin, Cardiovascular Center Grant 5520311 for I.J.B, supported this work.

REFERENCES

1. Hsu CY, McCulloch CE, Darbinian J, et al. Elevated blood pressure and risk of end-stage renal disease in subjects without baseline kidney disease. Arch Intern Med 2005;165:923–8.
2. Lawes CM, Vander Hoorn S, Rodgers A. Global burden of blood pressure-related disease, 2001. Lancet 2008;371:1513–8.

3. Lewington S, Clarke R, Qizilbash N, et al. Age-specific relevance of usual blood pressure to vascular mortality: a meta-analysis of individual data for one million adults in 61 prospective studies. Lancet 2002;360:1903–13.

4. Burt VL, Whelton P, Roccella EJ, et al. Prevalence of hypertension in the US adult population. Results from the third national health and Nutrition Examination Survey, 1988–1991. Hypertension 1995;25:305–13.

5. Go AS, Mozaffarian D, Roger VL, et al. Executive summary: heart disease and stroke statistics—2013 update: a report from the American Heart Association. Circulation 2013;127:143–52.

6. Hajjar I, Kotchen TA. Trends in prevalence, awareness, treatment, and control of hypertension in the United States, 1988–2000. JAMA 2003;290:199–206.

7. Lloyd-Jones DM, Hong Y, Labarthe D, et al. Defining and setting national goals for cardiovascular health promotion and disease reduction: the American Heart Association's strategic Impact Goal through 2020 and beyond. Circulation 2010;121:586–613.

8. Lawes CM, Vander HS, Rodgers A. Global burden of blood-pressure-related disease, 2001. Lancet 2008; 371:1513–8.

9. Munroe GB, Rice PB, Bochud KM, et al. Genetic variants in novel pathways influence blood pressure and cardiovascular disease risk. Nature 2011;478: 103–9.

10. Poulter N, Khaw KT, Hopwood BE, et al. Blood pressure and its correlates in an African tribe in urban and rural environments. J Epidemiol Community Health 1984;38:181–5.

11. Brunner HR, Gavras H. Is the renin system necessary? Am J Med 1980;69:739–45.

12. Chong JX, Buckingham KJ, Jhangiani SN, et al. The genetic basis of mendelian phenotypes: discoveries, challenges, and opportunities. Am J Human Genetics 2015;97:199–215.

13. Choi M, Scholl UI, Ji W, et al. Genetic diagnosis by whole exome capture and massively parallel DNA sequencing. Proc Natl Acad Sci USA 2009;106: 19062.

14. Miall WE, Oldham PD. The hereditary factor in arterial blood-pressure. Br Med J 1963;1:75–80.

15. Levy D, DeStefano AL, Larson MG, et al. Evidence for a gene influencing blood pressure on chromosome 17. Genome scan linkage results for longitudinal blood pressure phenotypes in subjects from the Framingham heart study. Hypertension 2000;36: 477–83.

16. White PC, Dupont J, New MI, et al. A mutation in CYP11B1 (Arg-448—His) associated with steroid 11 beta-hydroxylase deficiency in Jews of Moroccan origin. J Clin Invest 1991;87:1664–7.

17. Rosler A, White PC. Mutations in human 11 beta-hydroxylase genes: 11 betahydroxylase deficiency in Jews of Morocco and corticosterone methyl-oxidase II deficiency in Jews of Iran. J Steroid Biochem Mol Biol 1993;45:99–106.

18. Lifton RP, Dluhy RG, Powers M, et al. A chimaeric 11 beta-hydroxylase/aldosterone synthase gene causes glucocorticoidremediable aldosteronism and human hypertension. Nature 1992;355:262–5.

19. Rich GM, Ulick S, Cook S, et al. Glucocorticoid-remediable aldosteronism in a large kindred: clinical spectrum and diagnosis using a characteristic biochemical phenotype. Ann Intern Med 1992;116: 813–20.

20. Wilson FH, Disse-Nicodeme S, Choate KA, et al. Human hypertension caused by mutations in WNK kinases. Science 2001;293:1107–12.

21. Disse-Nicodeme S, Achard JM, Desitter I, et al. A newlocus on chromosome 12p13.3 for pseudohypoaldosteronism type II, an autosomal dominant form of hypertension. Am J Hum Genet 2000;67: 302–10.

22. Boyden LM, Choi M, Choate KA, et al. Mutations in kelch-like 3 and cullin 3 cause hypertension and electrolyte abnormalities. Nature 2012;482: 98–102.

23. Mayan H, Munter G, Shaharabany M, et al. Hypercalciuria in familial hyperkalemia and hypertension accompanies hyperkalemia and precedes hypertension: description of a large family with the Q565E WNK4 mutation. J Clin Endocrinol Metab 2004;89:4025–30.

24. Louis-Dit-Picard H, Barc J, Trujillano D, et al. KLHL3 mutations cause familial hyperkalemic hypertension by impairing ion transport in the distal nephron. Nat Genet 2012;44:456–60. S1–3.

25. Shimkets RA, Warnock DG, Bositis CM, et al. Liddle's syndrome: heritable human hypertension caused by mutations in the beta subunit of the epithelial sodium channel. Cell 1994;79:407–14.

26. Hansson JH, Nelson-Williams C, Suzuki H, et al. Hypertension caused by a truncated epithelial sodium channel gamma subunit: genetic heterogeneity of Liddle syndrome. Nat Genet 1995;11:76–82.

27. Botero-Velez M, Curtis JJ, Warnock DG. Brief report: Liddle's syndrome revisited–a disorder of sodium reabsorption in the distal tubule. N Engl J Med 1994; 330:178–81.

28. Liddle GW, Island DP, Ney RL, et al. Nonpituitary neoplasms and Cushing's syndrome. Ectopic 'adrenocorticotropin' produced by nonpituitary neoplasms as a cause of Cushing's syndrome. Arch Intern Med 1963;111:471–5.

29. Goldsmith O, Solomon DH, Horton R. Hypogonadism and mineralocorticoid excess. The 17-hydroxylase deficiency syndrome. N Engl J Med 1967;277: 673–7.

30. Imai T, Yanase T, Waterman MR, et al. Canadian Mennonites and individuals residing in the Friesland region of The Netherlands share the same molecular

basis of 17 alpha-hydroxylase deficiency. Hum Genet 1992;89:95–6.

31. Mune T, Rogerson FM, Nikkila H, et al. Human hypertension caused by mutations in the kidney isozyme of 11 beta-hydroxysteroid dehydrogenase. Nat Genet 1995;10:394–9.

32. Choi M, Scholl UI, Yue P, et al. K+ channel mutations in adrenal aldosterone-producing adenomas and hereditary hypertension. Science 2011;331:768–72.

33. Lifton RP. Molecular genetics of human blood pressure variation. Science 1996;272:676–80.

34. Lifton RP, Gharavi AG, Geller DS. Molecular mechanisms of human hypertension. Cell 2001;104:545–56.

35. Lifton RP. Genetic dissection of human blood pressure variation: common pathways from rare phenotypes. Harvey Lect 2004;100:71–101.

36. Keramati AR, Fathzadeh M, Go GW, et al. A form of the metabolic syndrome associated with mutations in DYRK1B. N Engl J Med 2014;370:1909–19.

37. Wellcome Trust Case Control Consortium. Genomewide association study of 14,000 cases of seven common diseases and 3,000 shared controls. Nature 2007;447:661–78.

38. Ho JE, Levy D, Rose L, et al. Discovery and replication of novel blood pressure genetic loci in the Women's Genome Health Study. J Hypertens 2011;29:62–9.

39. Takeuchi F, Isono M, Katsuya T, et al. Blood pressure and hypertension are associated with 7 loci in the Japanese population. Circulation 2010;121:2302–9.

40. Ehret GB, Munroe PB, Rice KM, et al. Genetic variants in novel pathways influence blood pressure and cardiovascular disease risk. Nature 2011;478:103–9.

41. Newton-Cheh C, Johnson T, Gateva V, et al. Genomewide association study identifies eight loci associated with blood pressure. Nat Genet 2009;41:666–76.

42. Tomaszewski M, Debiec R, Braund PS, et al. Genetic architecture of ambulatory blood pressure in the general population: insights from cardiovascular gene-centric array. Hypertension 2010;56:1069–76.

43. Newton-Cheh C, Larson MG, Vasan RS, et al. Association of common variants in NPPA and NPPB with circulating natriuretic peptides and blood pressure. Nat Genet 2009;41:348–53.

44. Johnson T, Gaunt TR, Newhouse SJ, et al. Blood pressure loci identified with a gene-centric array. Am J Hum Genet 2011;89:688–700.

45. Johnson AD, Newton-Cheh C, Chasman DI, et al. Association of hypertension drug target genes with blood pressure and hypertension in 86,588 individuals. Hypertension 2011;57:903–10.

46. Takeuchi F, Yamamoto K, Katsuya T, et al. Reevaluation of the association of seven candidate genes with blood pressure and hypertension: a replication study and meta-analysis with a larger sample size. Hypertens Res 2012;35(8):825–31.

47. Kato N, Takeuchi F, Tabara Y, et al. Meta-analysis of genome-wide association studies identifies common variants associated with blood pressure variation in east Asians. Nat Genet 2011;43:531–8.

48. Wain LV, Verwoert GC, O'Reilly PF, et al. Genomewide association study identifies six new loci influencing pulse pressure and mean arterial pressure. Nat Genet 2011;43:1005–11.

49. Levy D, Ehret GB, Rice K, et al. Genome-wide association study of blood pressure and hypertension. Nat Genet 2009;41:677–87.

50. Salvi E, Kutalik Z, Glorioso N, et al. Genomewide association study using a highdensity single nucleotide polymorphism array and case-control design identifies a novel essential hypertension susceptibility locus in the promoter region of endothelial NO synthase. Hypertension 2012;59:248–55.

51. Geller DS, Farhi A, Pinkerton N, et al. Activating mineralocorticoid receptor mutation in hypertension exacerbated by pregnancy. Science 2000;289:119–23.

52. Tabara Y, Kohara K, Kita Y, et al. Common variants in the ATP2B1 gene are associated with susceptibility to hypertension: the Japanese Millennium Genome Project. Hypertension 2010;56:973–80.

53. Lin Y, Lai X, Chen B, et al. Genetic variations in CYP17A1, CACNB2 and PLEKHA7 are associated with blood pressure and/or hypertension in She ethnic minority of China. Atherosclerosis 2011;219:709–14.

54. Hong KW, Jin HS, Lim JE, et al. Recapitulation of two genomewide association studies on blood pressure and essential hypertension in the Korean population. J Hum Genet 2010;55:336–41.

55. Ehret GB, O'Connor AA, Weder A, et al. Follow-up of a major linkage peak on chromosome 1 reveals suggestive QTLs associated with essential hypertension: GenNet study. Eur J Hum Genet 2009;17:1650–7.

56. Cho YS, Go MJ, Kim YJ, et al. A large-scale genome-wide association study of Asian populations uncovers genetic factors influencing eight quantitative traits. Nat Genet 2009;41:527–34.

57. Hong KW, Go MJ, Jin HS, et al. Genetic variations in ATP2B1, CSK, ARSG and CSMD1 loci are related to blood pressure and/or hypertension in two Korean cohorts. J Hum Hypertens 2010;24:367–72.

58. Fox ER, Young JH, Li Y, et al. Association of genetic variation with systolic and diastolic blood pressure among African Americans: the Candidate Gene Association Resource study. Hum Mol Genet 2011;20:2273–84.

59. Padmanabhan S, Melander O, Johnson T, et al. Genome-wide association study of blood pressure extremes identifies variant near UMOD associated with hypertension. PLoS Genet 2010;6:e1001177.

60. Manolio TA, Collins FS, Cox NJ, et al. Finding the missing heritability of complex diseases. Nature 2009;461:747–53.

61. Lango Allen H, Estrada K, Lettre G, et al. Hundreds of variants clustered in genomic loci and biological pathways affect human height. Nature 2010;467:832–8.

The Effects of Dietary Factors on Blood Pressure

Lawrence J. Appel, MD, MPH

KEYWORDS

- Blood pressure • Dietary factors • Hypertension • Cardiovascular disease • Renal disease

KEY POINTS

- A compelling body of evidence supports the concept that multiple dietary factors affect blood pressure (BP).
- Dietary changes that effectively lower BP are weight loss, reduced sodium intake, increased potassium intake, moderation of alcohol intake (among those who drink), and Dietary Approaches to Stop Hypertension (DASH)-style and vegetarian dietary patterns.
- In view of the increasing levels of BP in children and adults and the continuing epidemic of BP-related cardiovascular (CV) and renal diseases, efforts to reduce BP in both nonhypertensive and hypertensive individuals are warranted.
- The challenge to health care providers, researchers, government officials, and the general public is developing and implementing effective clinical and public health strategies that lead to sustained dietary changes among individuals and more broadly among whole populations.

INTRODUCTION

Elevated BP remains an extraordinarily common and important risk factor for CV and kidney diseases throughout the world.[1] According to the 2011 to 2012 National Health and Nutrition Examination Survey (NHANES), approximately 70 million adult Americans (29%) have hypertension (a systolic BP $\geq$140 mm Hg, a diastolic BP $\geq$90 mm Hg, or treatment with antihypertensive medication),[2] and at least as many Americans have prehypertension (systolic BP 120–139 mm Hg or diastolic BP 80–89 mm Hg, not on medication). Regrettably, the prevalence of hypertension has remained essentially unchanged for the past 2 decades, and control rates remain low, at approximately 53%.[3]

Systolic BP progressively rises with age, such that hypertension becomes almost ubiquitous among the elderly. As a result of the age-related rise in systolic BP, approximately 90% of adult Americans develop hypertension over their lifetime.[4] Elevated BP afflicts both men and women. African Americans, on average, have higher BP than non–African Americans as well as an increased risk of BP-related disease, in particular stroke and kidney disease.

BP is a strong, consistent, continuous, independent, and etiologically relevant risk factor for CV disease and renal disease.[5] Importantly, there is no evidence of a BP threshold, that is, the risk of CV disease increases progressively throughout the range of usual BP, including the prehypertensive range.[6] It has been estimated that approximately a third of BP-related deaths from coronary heart disease (CHD) occur in individuals with BP in the nonhypertensive range. Accordingly, prehypertensive individuals not only have a high probability of developing hypertension but also carry an excess risk of CV disease compared with those with a normal BP (systolic BP <120 mm Hg and diastolic BP <80 mm Hg).[7] Approximately 54% of strokes and 47% of ischemic heart disease events worldwide have been attributed to an elevated BP.[8]

Elevated BP results from environmental factors (including dietary factors), genetic factors, and

Text adapted from Appel LJ, Brands MW, Daniels SR, et al. Dietary approaches to prevent and treat hypertension: a scientific statement from the American Heart Association. Hypertension 2006;47(2):296–308.
Welch Center for Prevention, Epidemiology, and Clinical Research, Johns Hopkins University, 2024 East Monument Street, Suite 2-642, Baltimore, MD 21205-2223, USA
E-mail address: lappel@jhmi.edu

cardiology.theclinics.com

interactions among these factors. Of the environmental factors that affect BP (diet, physical inactivity, toxins, and psychosocial factors), diet likely has a predominant role in BP homeostasis. Well-established dietary modifications that lower BP are a reduced sodium intake, weight loss, moderation of alcohol consumption (among those who drink excessively), and healthy dietary patterns, specifically, Dietary Approaches to Stop Hypertension (DASH)-style diets, vegetarian diets, and, to a lesser extent, Mediterranean-style diets.

In nonhypertensive individuals, dietary changes that lower BP have the potential to prevent hypertension and reduce the risk of BP-related CV disease. Even an apparently small BP reduction, if applied broadly to an entire population, could have an enormous, beneficial impact. For example, it has been estimated that a 3 mm Hg average reduction in systolic BP could lead to an 8% reduction in stroke mortality and a 5% reduction in mortality from CHD (**Fig. 1**).[9] In uncomplicated stage I hypertension (systolic BP 140–159 mm Hg or diastolic BP 90–99 mm Hg), dietary changes can serve as first-line therapy, before antihypertensive medication. Among hypertensive individuals who are already on medication, dietary changes can further lower BP and make it possible to reduce the number and doses of medications. In general, the magnitude of BP reduction from dietary changes is greater in hypertensive individuals than in nonhypertensive individuals.

Although dietary changes lower BP, there is considerably less evidence on whether dietary changes blunt the age-related rise in systolic BP. On average, systolic BP rises by approximately 0.6 mm Hg per year. Efforts to prevent this age-associated rise in systolic BP hold the greatest promise as a means to prevent elevated BP and curb the epidemic of BP-related disease. Unfortunately, even the longest diet-BP intervention trials have lasted less than 5 years. Whether the

BP reductions observed in these trials have merely shifted the age-associated rise in BP curve downward, without a change in slope (**Fig. 2**), or actually reduced its slope (see **Fig. 2**) cannot be determined. Still, evidence from migration studies, ecologic studies, and, most recently, observational analyses of trial data[10] suggest that dietary factors should reduce the rise in systolic BP with age.

The objective of this article is to synthesize evidence on the relationship of diet and BP. The summary of evidence and corresponding recommendations largely reflect previous reviews.[11,12]

DIETARY FACTORS THAT REDUCE BLOOD PRESSURE
Weight Loss

Weight is directly associated with BP. The importance of this relationship is reinforced by the high and increasing prevalence of obesity throughout the world. In the United States, approximately 69% of adults have a body mass index (BMI) greater than or equal to 25 kg/m^2 and, therefore, are classified as either overweight or obese; approximately 35% of adults are obese (BMI $\geq$30 kg/m^2).[13] Likewise, among infants, toddlers, children, and adolescents, the prevalence of high weight persists, with scant evidence of any improvement.

Weight loss lowers BP. Reductions in BP occur before, and even without, attainment of a desirable body weight. In a meta-analysis of 25 trials, an average weight loss of 5.1 kg reduced systolic BP by a mean of 4.4 mm Hg and diastolic BP by a mean of 3.6 mm Hg.[14] In subgroup analyses, BP reductions were greater in those who lost more weight. Dose-response analyses[15] and observational studies also provide evidence that greater weight loss leads to greater BP reduction. Given the potential for huge reductions in weight, however, a linear dose-response relationship is unlikely.

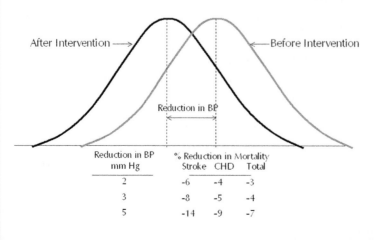

Fig. 1. Estimated effects of population-wide shifts in systolic BP on mortality. CHD, coronary heart disease. (*Data from* Stamler R. Implications of the INTERSALT study. Hypertension 1991;17(1 Suppl):I16–20.)

Reduction in BP mm Hg	% Reduction in Mortality		
	Stroke	CHD	Total
2	-6	-4	-3
3	-8	-5	-4
5	-14	-9	-7

Reduction in BP

After Intervention →   ←Before Intervention

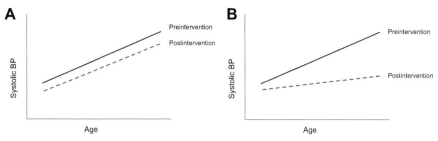

Fig. 2. (*A*) Model in which a dietary intervention shifts age-BP curve downward without affecting slope. (*B*) Model in which a dietary intervention that shifts age-BP curve downward and reduces its slope.

Other research has documented that modest weight loss, with or without sodium reduction, can prevent hypertension by approximately 20% among overweight, nonhypertensive individuals and can facilitate the reduction of the number and doses of medications. Behavioral intervention trials have uniformly achieved short-term weight loss, primarily through a reduction in energy intake. In several instances, substantial weight loss has also been maintained over 3 or more years.[16–18] Regular physical activity is well recognized as a critical factor in sustaining weight loss. Whether weight loss can blunt the age-related rise in systolic BP is uncertain. In 1 of the longest weight loss trials, those individuals who sustained a greater than 10 kg weight loss achieved a lower BP that nonetheless rose over time (**Fig. 3**).[15]

In aggregate, available evidence strongly supports weight reduction as an effective approach to lower BP.

Reduced Salt (Sodium Chloride) Intake

On average, as dietary sodium intake rises, so does BP. Available types of evidence include animal studies, epidemiologic studies, dose-

response trials, and meta-analyses of trials. To date, more than 100 randomized trials have been performed. In one of the most recent meta-analyses,[19] a reduction in sodium intake of 2.3 g/d lowered systolic BP by 3.8 mm Hg in adults; larger BP reductions occurred in older persons compared with younger persons, blacks compared with whites, and hypertensive individuals compared with normotensive individuals. In a small but well-done trial of patients with medication-treated, resistant hypertension, reducing sodium intake by approximately 4.5 g/d lowered systolic/diastolic BP by 22.7/9.1 mm Hg.[20]

The most persuasive evidence on the effects of sodium intake on BP comes from rigorously controlled, dose-response studies.[21,22] Each of these trials tested at least 3 sodium levels, and each documented statistically significant, direct, progressive, dose-response relationships. The largest of these trials, the DASH-Sodium trial, tested the effects of 3 different sodium intakes separately in 2 diets—the DASH diet (discussed later) and a control diet more typical of what Americans usually eat. As estimated from 24-hour urine collections, the 3 sodium levels (lower, intermediate, and higher) provided 65 mmol/d, 107

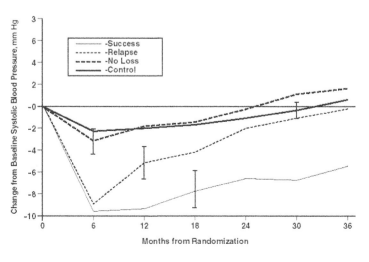

Fig. 3. Mean systolic BP change in the Trials of Hypertension Prevention, phase II (TOHP2) in 4 groups of participants: those assigned to weight loss group who successfully maintained weight loss, those assigned to weight loss group who lost weight but experienced relapse, those assigned to weight loss group who never lost weight, and control group. (*From* Stevens VJ, Obarzanek E, Cook NR, et al. Long-term weight loss and changes in blood pressure: results of the Trials of Hypertension Prevention, phase II. Ann Intern Med 2001;134(1):8; with permission.)

mmol/d, and 142 mmol/d of sodium, respectively (corresponding to 1.5 g/d, 2.5 g/d, and 3.3 g/d).

The main results of this trial are displayed in **Fig. 4**. The BP response to sodium reduction, although direct and progressive, was nonlinear. Decreasing sodium intake by approximately 0.9 g/d (40 mmol/d) caused a greater BP reduction when the starting sodium intake was below 100 mmol/d than when it was above this level. In subgroup analyses of this trial,[23,24] a reduced sodium intake significantly lowered BP in each of the major subgroups studied (ie, African American, non-African American, men, and women). Sodium reduction significantly lowered BP in nonhypertensive individuals on both diets.

In addition to lowering BP, trials have documented that a reduced sodium intake can prevent hypertension (relative risk reduction of approximately 20% with or without concomitant weight loss), can lower BP even in the setting of BP-lowering medications,[25] and can improve hypertension control. In observational studies, a low sodium intake is associated with a blunted age-related rise in systolic BP. Several observational studies have explored the relationship of sodium intake with CV disease. These reports have been notable for their inconsistent and occasionally paradoxic results,[26,27] which likely result from methodological limitations, in particular, the potential for reverse causality and the challenge of accurately estimating usual sodium intake.[28]

To date, few trials have reported the effects of a reduced sodium intake on clinical CV events.[25,26,29] Two trials tested reduced sodium lifestyle interventions, and 1 trial assessed the effects of a reduced sodium/high potassium salt substitute. In each, there was a 21% to 41% reduction in clinical CV disease events in those who received the reduced sodium intervention (significant reduction in 2 studies[26,29]). A fourth trial with few CVD outcomes had a null result. In a meta-analysis of these trials, there was a 20% reduction in CVD outcomes.[30] Hence, direct evidence from trials, albeit limited, is consistent with indirect evidence on the health benefits of sodium reduction.[31]

Similar to other interventions, the BP response to changes in dietary sodium intake is heterogeneous. Despite attempts to classify individuals in research studies as salt sensitive and salt resistant, the change in BP in response to a change in sodium intake is not binary.[32] Rather, the change in BP from a reduced sodium intake has a continuous distribution, that is, individuals have greater or lesser degrees of BP reduction. In general, the extent of BP reduction as a result of reduced sodium intake is greater in blacks, middle-aged and older-aged persons, and individuals with hypertension and likely those with diabetes or kidney disease. These groups tend to have a less-responsive renin-angiotensin-aldosterone system.[33] It has been hypothesized that sodium sensitivity is a phenotype that reflects subclinical kidney dysfunction.[34] As discussed later, genetic and dietary factors also influence the response to sodium. The rise in BP for a given increase in sodium is blunted in the setting of either the DASH diet or a high dietary potassium intake.

A reduced sodium intake should have other beneficial effects that are independent of its effects on BP. Potential benefits include a reduced risk of subclinical CVD (ie, left ventricular hypertrophy, ventricular fibrosis, and diastolic dysfunction), kidney damage, gastric cancer, and disordered mineral metabolism (ie, increased urinary calcium excretion, potentially leading to osteoporosis).[35] Specifically, in cross-sectional studies, left ventricular mass is directly related to sodium intake, and 1 small trial in the early 1990s documented that sodium reduction can reduce left ventricular mass.

There is no convincing or consistent evidence of harm from a reduced sodium intake. Although some sodium intake is essential, there is no evidence that inadequate sodium intake is a public health problem. Extreme sodium reduction to less than 20 mmol/d might adversely affect blood lipids and insulin resistance; however, moderate sodium reduction has no such effects.[36,37] A potential adverse effect of a reduced sodium intake is an increase in plasma renin activity (PRA) and uric acid. In contrast to the well-accepted benefits of BP reduction, however, the clinical relevance of modest

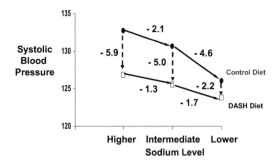

Fig. 4. Mean systolic BP changes in the DASH-Sodium trial. The sample size was 412; 59% were prehypertensive and 57% were African American. Solid lines display the effects of sodium reduction in the 2 diets; hatched lines display the effects of the DASH diet at each sodium level. (*Adapted from* Sacks FM, Svetkey LP, Vollmer WM, et al. Effects on blood pressure of reduced dietary sodium and the Dietary Approaches to Stop Hypertension (DASH) diet. DASH-Sodium Collaborative Research Group. N Engl J Med 2001;344(1):6; with permission.)

rises in PRA and uric acid as a result of sodium reduction and other antihypertensive therapies is uncertain. Thiazide diuretics, a class of antihypertensive drug therapies that raises PRA and uric acid, substantially reduces CV disease risk.[38]

Available evidence supports population-wide sodium reduction, as recommended by the professional, national and international guidelines for Americans and numerous other organizations. Current dietary guidelines recommend an upper limit of 2300 mg/d in the general population and an upper limit of 1500 mg/d in blacks, middle-age and older-aged persons, and individuals with hypertension, diabetes, or chronic kidney disease (CKD); together these groups represent well over 50% of US adults.[39] In this setting, the American Heart Association set 1.5 g/d (65 mmol/d) of sodium as the recommended upper limit of intake for all Americans.[40] Survey data indicate that most children and adults exceed this limit.

In summary, available data strongly support current, population-wide recommendations to lower sodium intake. Consumers should choose foods low in sodium and limit the amount of sodium added to food. Because more than 75% of consumed sodium comes from processed foods, however, any meaningful strategy to reduce sodium intake must involve food manufacturers and restaurants. Recent guidelines have recommended that the food industry should progressively reduce the sodium added to foods by 50% over 10 years.[41] In the absence of meaningful reductions in sodium intake through voluntary recommendations, a recent Institute of Medicine report has recommended a national approach, implemented through the Food and Drug Administration, to accomplish population-wide reductions in sodium intake.[42]

Increased Potassium Intake

High potassium intake is associated with lower BP. Available evidence includes animal studies, observational studies, clinical trials, and meta-analyses of these trials. Although data from individual trials have typically been inconsistent, several meta-analyses have each documented a significant inverse relationship between potassium intake and BP in hypertensive patients and equivocal effects in nonhypertensive individuals.[43] In 1 meta-analysis, a net increase in urinary potassium excretion of 2 g/d (50 mmol/d) was associated with average systolic and diastolic BP reductions of 4.4 mm Hg and 2.5 mm Hg, respectively, in hypertensive individuals and 1.8 mm Hg and 1.0 mm Hg, respectively, in nonhypertensive persons. Increased potassium has beneficial effects on BP in the setting of a low potassium intake

(eg, 1.3–1.4 g/d or 35–40 mmol/d) or a much higher intake (eg, 3.3 g/d or 84 mmol/d).[44] Increased potassium intake reduces BP to a greater extent in blacks compared with whites and, therefore, may be a valuable tool to reduce health disparities related to elevated BP and its complications.

Because a high intake of potassium can be achieved through diet and because potassium contained in foods is also accompanied by a variety of other nutrients, the preferred strategy to increase potassium intake is to consume foods, such as fruits and vegetables that are rich in potassium. In the DASH trial, the 2 groups that increased fruit and vegetable consumption both lowered BP.[45] The DASH diet provides approximately 4.7 g/d (120 mmol/d) of potassium. Another trial documented that increased fruit and vegetable intake lowers BP, but it did not specify the amount of potassium that was provided.[46]

Potassium and sodium interact such that the effects of potassium on BP depend on the concurrent intake of sodium and vice versa. Specifically, an increased intake of potassium has greater BP-lowering effects in the setting of a higher sodium intake and lesser BP effects when sodium intake is already low. Conversely, the BP reduction from a lower sodium intake is greatest when potassium intake is also low. In 1 trial, a high potassium intake (120 mmol/d) blunted the pressor response to increased sodium intake in nonhypertensive black men and to a lesser extent in nonblacks (**Fig. 5**).[47] A 2 × 2 factorial trial,

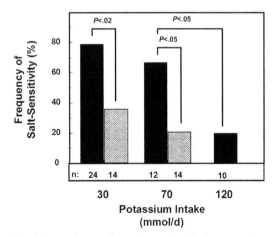

Fig. 5. Prevalence of sodium sensitivity in normotensive individuals (blacks, solid bars; whites, crosshatched bars) at 3 levels of potassium intake. Sodium sensitivity is defined by a sodium-induced increase in mean arterial pressure of at least 3 mm Hg. (*From* Morris RC Jr, Sebastian A, Forman A, et al. Normotensive salt sensitivity: effects of race and dietary potassium. Hypertension 1999;33(1):20; with permission.)

conducted in Australia, tested the effects of reduced sodium intake and increased potassium intake, alone or together, on BP in 212 hypertensive individuals; in this trial, a reduced sodium intake lowered BP to the same extent as an increased potassium intake; however, the combination did not further lower BP. Overall, available data are consistent with subadditive effects of reduced sodium intake and increased potassium intake on BP.

The dearth of dose-response studies precludes a firm recommendation for a specific level of potassium intake to lower BP. An Institute of Medicine committee, however, set the recommended potassium intake level at 4.7 g/d (120 mmol/d).[48] This level is similar to the average total potassium intake in clinical trials, the highest dose in the 1 available dose-response trial, and the potassium content of the DASH diet.[45]

In the generally healthy population with normal kidney function, a potassium intake from foods above 4.7 g/d (120 mmol/d) poses no risk because excess potassium is readily excreted. In individuals whose urinary potassium excretion is impaired, however, an intake less than 4.7 g/d (120 mmol/d) is appropriate, because of adverse cardiac effects (dysrhythmias) from hyperkalemia. Common drugs that impair potassium excretion are angiotensin-converting enzyme inhibitors, angiotensin receptor blockers, nonsteroidal anti-inflammatory drugs, and potassium-sparing diuretics. Medical conditions associated with impaired renal excretion of potassium include diabetes, CKD, end-stage renal disease, severe heart failure, and adrenal insufficiency. Elderly individuals are at increased risk of hyperkalemia. Available evidence is insufficient to identify the level of kidney function at which individuals with CKD are at risk for hyperkalemia from a high dietary intake of potassium. In this setting, namely, patients with advanced CKD, that is, stage 3 or 4, an expert panel set a wide range of recommended potassium intake — 2000 mg/d to 4000 mg/d.[49]

Moderation of Alcohol Consumption

Observational and experimental studies have documented a direct, dose-response relationship between alcohol intake and BP, particularly as the intake of alcohol increases above 2 drinks per day.[50] This relationship is independent of potential confounders, such as age, obesity, and sodium intake.[51] Although some studies have shown that the alcohol-BP relationship also extends into the light drinking range, that is, at or below 2 drinks per day, this is the range in which alcohol may reduce the risk of CHD.

A meta-analysis of 15 randomized trials reported that decreased alcohol consumption (median reduction in self-reported alcohol intake of 76%, range 16% to 100%) lowered BP by 3.3/2.0 mm Hg.[50] Reductions were similar in nonhypertensives and hypertensive individuals, and the relationship seemed dose-dependent.

In aggregate, available evidence supports moderation of alcohol intake (among those who drink) as an effective strategy to lower BP. The prevailing consensus is that alcohol consumption should be limited to no more than 2 alcoholic drinks per day in men and to no more than 1 alcoholic drink per day in women and lighter weight persons (1 drink [providing ~ 15 gm of alcohol] is defined as 12 oz of regular beer, 5 oz of wine [12% alcohol], and 1.5 oz of 80-proof distilled spirits).

Dietary Patterns

Vegetarian diets

Certain dietary patterns, in particular vegetarian diets, have been associated with low BP. In industrialized countries, where elevated BP is commonplace, individuals who consume a vegetarian diet have markedly lower BP than nonvegetarians. Some of the lowest BPs observed in industrialized countries have been documented in strict vegetarians living in Massachusetts. Vegetarians may also experience a slower age-related rise in BP.

Several aspects of a vegetarian lifestyle might affect BP. These lifestyle factors include nondietary factors (eg, physical activity), established dietary risk factors (eg, sodium, potassium, weight, and alcohol), and other aspects of a vegetarian diet (eg, high fiber and no meat). To a limited extent, observational studies have controlled for the well-established dietary determinants of BP. For instance, in a study of Seventh-day Adventists, analyses were adjusted for weight but not dietary sodium or potassium intake.[52] In a recent meta-analysis of 7 trials and 32 cohort studies, vegetarian diets were associated with lower systolic BP (mean net difference of −6.9 mm Hg) and diastolic BP (mean net difference of −4.7 mm Hg) compared with omnivorous diets.[53]

The Dietary Approaches to Stop Hypertension diet

The DASH trial was a randomized feeding study that tested the effects of 3 diets on BP.[45] The most effective diet, now termed the DASH diet, emphasized fruits, vegetables, and low-fat dairy products; included whole grains, poultry, fish, and nuts; and was reduced in fats, red meat, sweets, and sugar-containing beverages. It was rich in potassium, magnesium, calcium, and fiber and reduced in total fat, saturated fat, and cholesterol; it was also slightly increased in protein. Among all participants, the DASH diet significantly lowered BP by a mean of 5.5/3.0 mm Hg, each net of control. The BP-lowering effects of the diets were rapid, occurring within only 2 weeks (**Fig. 6**).

In subgroup analyses,[45] the DASH diet significantly lowered BP in all major subgroups (men, women, African Americans, non–African Americans, hypertensive individuals, and nonhypertensives). The effects of the DASH diet, however, in the African American participants were striking (mean net BP reductions of 6.9/3.7 mm Hg) and were significantly greater than corresponding reductions in white participants (net BP reductions of 3.3/2.4 mm Hg). The effects in hypertensive individuals (net BP reductions of 11.6/5.3 mm Hg) have obvious clinical significance. The corresponding effects in nonhypertensive individuals (3.5/2.2 mm Hg) have major public health importance (see **Fig. 1**). In a subsequent trial that enrolled a similar population,[21] the DASH diet significantly lowered BP at each of 3 sodium levels (see **Fig. 4**), and the combination of the DASH diet with sodium reduction resulted in the lowest level of BP.

The issue of whether modifying macronutrient content might improve the DASH diet was tested in a third trial, Optimal Macronutrient Intake Trial to Prevent Heart Disease (OmniHeart).[54] This feeding study tested 3 variants of the DASH diets (a diet rich in carbohydrate [58% of total calories] and similar to the original DASH diet, a second diet rich in protein [approximately half from plant sources], and a third diet rich in unsaturated fat [predominantly monounsaturated fat]). In several respects, each diet was similar to the original DASH diet — each was reduced in saturated fat, cholesterol, and sodium and rich in fruit, vegetables, fiber, and potassium at recommended levels. Although each diet lowered systolic BP (**Fig. 7**), substituting some of the carbohydrate (approximately 10% of total kcal) with either protein (approximately half from plant sources) or with unsaturated fat (mostly monounsaturated fat) further lowered BP.

Speculation about the effective components of DASH-style diets has been considerable. The diet that emphasized fruits and vegetables resulted in BP reductions that were approximately half of the total effect of the DASH diet (see **Fig. 6**). Fruits and vegetables are rich in potassium, magnesium, fiber, and many other nutrients. Of these nutrients, potassium is best established to lower BP, particularly in hypertensive individuals and in African Americans. In view of the additional BP reduction from the DASH diet beyond that of the fruits and vegetables diet, some other aspect(s) of the DASH diet further lowered BP. Compared with the fruits and vegetables diet, the DASH diet had more vegetables, low-fat dairy products, and fish and was lower in red meat, sugar, and refined carbohydrates.

The DASH diet is safe and broadly applicable to the general population. Because of its relatively high potassium, phosphorus, and protein content, however, this diet is not recommended for persons with advanced CKD.[49]

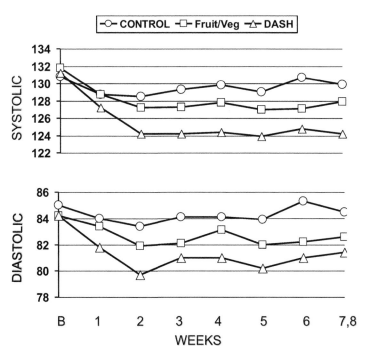

Fig. 6. BP by week during the DASH feeding study in 3 diets (control diet, fruits and vegetables diet, and the DASH diet). (*Adapted from* Appel LJ, Moore TJ, Obarzanek E, et al. A clinical trial of the effects of dietary patterns on blood pressure. DASH Collaborative Research Group. N Engl J Med 1997;336(16):1117–24.)

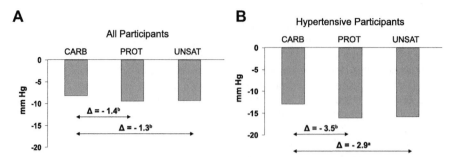

Fig. 7. Effects of 3 healthy dietary patterns tested in the OmniHeart feeding study on systolic BP (CARB [similar to the DASH diet], PROT [rich in protein, approximately half from plant sources], UNSAT [rich in monounsaturated fat]) (A) in all participants and (B) in hypertensive participants. [a] P<.05; [b] P<.01. (*Adapted from* Appel LJ, Sacks FM, Carey VJ, et al. Effects of protein, monounsaturated fat, and carbohydrate intake on blood pressure and serum lipids: results of the OmniHeart randomized trial. JAMA 2005;294(19):2455–64.)

Mediterranean diets

Mediterranean diet is a general descriptive term applied to diets consumed in several regions close to the Mediterranean Sea. Typically, these diets are rich in plant foods (fruit, vegetables, breads, other forms of cereals, potatoes, beans, nuts, and seeds). Fruit is the typical daily dessert, and olive oil is the principal source of fat. Dairy products (mostly cheese and yogurt), fish, and poultry are consumed in low to moderate amounts, 0 to 4 eggs are consumed weekly, red meat is consumed in low amounts, and wine is consumed in low to moderate amounts, usually with meals. This diet is low in saturated fat (≤7%–8% of energy) but moderate to high in total fat, ranging from less than 25% to greater than 40% of energy. Such a diet is similar to the DASH-style diet, termed UNSAT, tested in the OmniHeart.[54]

In observational studies, Mediterranean diets are associated with a reduced risk of CV disease and other degenerative conditions.[55] In a major trial, Prevención con Dieta Mediterránea (PREDIMED), advice to consume a Mediterranean diet coupled with supplemental foods (either extra-virgin olive oil or mixed nuts) reduced the risk of CV disease, in particular stroke, an outcome that largely reflects BP.[56] Still, the effects of a Mediterranean style diet on BP seem to be modest, that is, net reductions in systolic and diastolic BP less than 2 mm Hg, in a meta-analysis of 6 trials.[57]

DIETARY FACTORS WITH LIMITED OR UNCERTAIN EFFECTS
Fish Oil Supplementation

Several predominantly small trials and meta-analyses of these trials have documented that high-dose, omega-3 polyunsaturated fatty acid (commonly termed fish oil) supplements can reduce BP in hypertensive individuals.[58] In nonhypertensive individuals, BP reductions tend to be small or nonsignificant. In some analyses, the effects seem dose-dependent, with BP reductions occurring at high doses of fish oil, namely, 3 g/d or more. In hypertensive individuals, average BP reductions were 2.6/1.5 mm Hg. Side effects, including a fishy taste and belching, are common. In view of these side effects and the high dose required to lower BP, fish oil supplements cannot be routinely recommended to lower BP.

Fiber

Fiber consists of the indigestible components of food from plants. Evidence from observational studies and several trials suggests that increased fiber intake may reduce BP. More than 20 trials of fiber supplementation have been conducted. Most did not have BP as their primary outcome, and many had a multicomponent intervention. Also differences in definition and classification of fiber have complicated interpretation of trial findings. Two meta-analyses estimated the impact of fiber supplements on BP,[59,60] and both noted net systolic and diastolic BP reductions less than 2 mm Hg, often nonsignificant. Overall, data are insufficient to recommend supplemental fiber or an increased intake of dietary fiber alone to lower BP.

Calcium and Magnesium

Evidence that increased dietary calcium intake might lower BP comes from a variety of sources, including animal studies, observational studies, trials, and meta-analyses. In a 1995 meta-analysis of 23 observational studies, Cappuccio and colleagues[61] noted an inverse association between dietary calcium intake and BP. The effect size was small, however, and there was evidence of publication bias and heterogeneity across studies. Subsequent meta-analyses of randomized trials documented modest reductions in BP of 0.9–1.4/0.2–0.8 mm Hg from calcium supplementation (400–2000 mg/d).[62] The level of dietary calcium intake may affect the pressor response to sodium. In 3 small trials, calcium supplementation mitigated the effects of a high sodium intake on BP.

Evidence implicating magnesium as a major determinant of BP is inconsistent. In observational studies, often cross-sectional, a common finding is an inverse association between dietary magnesium and BP, a relationship seen in a pooled analysis of 29 observational studies. In a meta-analysis of 20 randomized clinical trials, however, there was no clear effect of increased magnesium intake on BP.[63]

Overall, evidence is insufficient to recommend either supplemental calcium or magnesium to lower BP.

Intake of Fats Other than Omega-3 Polyunsaturated Fatty Acid

Total fat includes saturated fat, omega-3 polyunsaturated fat, omega-6 polyunsaturated fat, and monounsaturated fat. Early studies focused on the effects of total fat intake on BP. There is a plausible biological basis, however, to hypothesize that certain types of fat (eg, omega-3 polyunsaturated fat) might lower BP and that other types of fat (eg, saturated fat) might raise it.

Saturated fat
Several observational studies and a few trials have assessed the effects of saturated fat on BP. In the vast majority, including 2 prospective observational studies, the Nurses' Health Study and the Health Professionals Follow-up Study, saturated fat intake was not associated with incident hypertension. In the few available clinical trials, diet interventions focused on reducing saturated fat had no effect on BP. Because most trials tested diets that were simultaneously reduced in saturated fat and increased in polyunsaturated fat, the absence of a BP effect also suggests no benefit from polyunsaturated fat.

Omega-6 polyunsaturated fat intake
Dietary intake of omega-6 polyunsaturated fat (mainly linoleic acid in Western diets) has little or no effect on BP. In an overview of cross-sectional studies that correlated BP with tissue or blood levels of omega-6 polyunsaturated fat, there was no apparent relationship. Prospective observational studies and clinical trials have likewise been unsupportive.

Monounsaturated fat intake
Although the earliest trials did not support a relationship between monounsaturated fat and BP, subsequent trials have shown that diets rich in monounsaturated fats modestly lower BP.[64] An increase in monounsaturated fat, however, is commonly linked with a reduction in the amount of carbohydrate consumed, potentially with a change in the type of carbohydrate as well.[65] Hence, it remains unclear whether the effects of increased monounsaturated fat intake reflect an increase in this nutrient and/or a decrease in carbohydrate intake or change in the type of carbohydrate, per se.

Carbohydrate
Both amount and type of carbohydrate may affect BP, but the evidence is uncertain. Worldwide, many populations who eat carbohydrate-rich, low-fat diets have low BP levels compared with Western countries. Still, the results of observational studies have been inconsistent. In small early trials, increasing carbohydrate by reducing total fat typically did not reduce BP. In the Omni-Heart, partial substitution of carbohydrate with either protein (approximately half from plant sources) or monounsaturated fat lowered BP.[54] In a subsequent trial, a high–glycemic index diet compared with low–glycemic index diet had no significant effect on BP.[66]

An emerging but inconclusive body of evidence suggests that increased intake of added sugars might raise BP. Studies include animal studies in which rats are fed high doses of fructose, acute ingestion studies in which humans are fed high doses of different sugars, and more recently epidemiologic studies. In cross-sectional studies, higher sugar-sweetened beverage intake has been associated with elevated BP in adolescents. In prospective observational studies, consumption of more than 1 soft drink per day significantly increased the odds of developing high BP.[67] In post hoc analyses of a completed trial, there was a direct association between reductions in sugar-sweetened beverage intake with reductions in BP.[68] Nonetheless, results from randomized trials in humans are inconsistent.[69] Overall, additional research is warranted before making recommendations about the amount and type of carbohydrate as a means to lower BP.

Cholesterol

Few studies have examined the BP effects of dietary cholesterol. In the observational analyses of the Multiple Risk Factor Intervention Trial, there were significant, direct relationships between cholesterol intake (mg/d) and both systolic and diastolic BP. The Keys dietary lipid score (from an equation that includes intakes of dietary cholesterol as well as saturated fate and polyunsaturated fat) was also associated with diastolic BP but not systolic BP. In longitudinal analyses from the Chicago Western Electric Study,[70] there were significant positive relationships of change in systolic BP over 8 years with dietary cholesterol as well as the Keys score (Keys Score predicts the effects of dietary saturated fat, polunsaturated fat, and cholesterol on serum cholesterol).[59] Despite these reports, the paucity of evidence precludes any firm conclusion about a relationship between dietary cholesterol and BP.

Protein Intake

An extensive, and generally consistent, body of evidence from observational studies has documented inverse associations between BP and protein intake, in particular protein from plants. Two major observational studies, the International Study of Macro/Micronutrients and Blood Pressure (INTERMAP) and the Chicago Western Electric Study, have documented significant inverse relationships between protein intake and BP.[70,71] In these studies, protein from plant sources was associated with lower BP, whereas protein from animal sources had no significant effect.

In contrast to the large volume of evidence from observational studies, few trials have examined the effects of increased protein intake on BP. Two trials documented that increased protein intake from soy supplements can reduce BP. In 1 trial, supplemental soy protein (total of 25% kcal protein, 12.5% kcal from soy) lowered average 24-hour BP by 5.9/2.6 mm Hg in hypertensive individuals. In a large trial conducted in the People's Republic of China, supplemental soy protein, which increased total protein intake from 12% kcal to 16% kcal, lowered average BP by 4.3/2.7 mm Hg, net of a control group that received supplemental carbohydrate. A meta-analysis of 40 trials documented that supplementation of diet with protein, compared with carbohydrate, significantly lowered systolic BP by 1.8 mm Hg and diastolic BP by 1.2 mm Hg, with no difference in effects from animal and vegetable protein.[72] In aggregate, clinical trials and observational studies support the hypothesis that an increased intake of protein from plants can lower BP. Further evidence is needed, however, before recommendations can be made.

Vitamin C

Laboratory studies, depletion-repletion studies, and observational studies suggest that increased vitamin C intake and higher vitamin C levels are associated with lower BP. A large number of randomized trials, often with small samples, have tested whether vitamin C supplements lower BP. A 2012 meta-analysis of these trials suggested that supplementation of diet with vitamin C might lower BP.[73] At this time, it remains unclear whether an increased intake or supplementation of diet with vitamin C lowers BP.

GENE-DIET INTERACTIONS

A substantial and increasing body of evidence has documented that genetic factors affect BP levels and the BP response to dietary changes. Most of the available research has focused on genetic factors that influence the BP response to dietary sodium intake. Several genotypes that affect BP have been identified, and most influence the renin-angiotensin-aldosterone axis or renal sodium handling. In a line of research that has focused on mendelian diseases associated with either high or low BP, 6 genes associated with higher BP and 8 genes associated with lower BP have been identified.[74] Of considerable importance is that each of these genes regulates renal sodium handling—mutations that increase net sodium chloride reabsorption raise BP, whereas mutations that lower sodium chloride reabsorption reduce BP.

A few trials have examined the interactive effects of specific genotypes and the BP response to dietary changes. In trials, genetic variation of the angiotensinogen gene modified the BP response to changes in sodium intake in whites,[22] the BP response to weight change, and the DASH diet.[75] Polymorphism of the α-adducin gene also seems to affect the BP response to sodium chloride.[76] Lastly, angiotensin-converting enzyme insertion/deletion polymorphism may also affect the BP response to weight change.[77]

EFFECTS OF MULTIPLE DIETARY CHANGES

Despite the potential for large BP reductions from simultaneously implementing multiple dietary changes, few trials have examined the combined effects of multicomponent interventions. In general, multicomponent intervention trials have documented subadditivity, that is, the BP effect of interventions with 2 or more components is less than the sum of BP reductions from interventions that implement each component alone. Despite subadditivity, the BP effects of multicomponent interventions are often large and clinically relevant. One small but well-controlled trial tested the effects of a comprehensive program of supervised exercise with provision of prepared meals to accomplish weight loss, sodium reduction, and the DASH diet; participants were medication-treated hypertensive adults. The program substantially lowered daytime ambulatory BP by 12.1/6.6 mm Hg, net of control.[78] Subsequently, a behavioral intervention trial, PREMIER, tested the effects of the major lifestyle recommendations (weight loss, sodium reduction, increased physical activity, and the DASH diet).[79] In nonhypertensives, mean BP reductions were 9.2/5.8 mm Hg (3.1/2.0 mm Hg, net of control). In hypertensive individuals, none of whom were on medication, corresponding BP reductions were 14.2/7.4 mm Hg (6.3/3.6 mm Hg, net of control).

BEHAVIORAL INTERVENTIONS TO ACCOMPLISH LIFESTYLE MODIFICATION

Numerous behavioral intervention trials have tested the BP effects of dietary change. Several theories and models have informed the design of these trials, including social cognitive theory, self-applied behavior modification techniques, behavioral self-management, the relapse prevention model, and the transtheoretic or stages-of-change model. Application of these theories and models typically leads to a common intervention approach that emphasizes behavioral skills training, self-monitoring, self-regulation, and motivational interviewing. Often these studies enrolled motivated individuals, selected in part because of their self-reported readiness to change. Furthermore, these studies relied on skilled therapists, often health educators or dietitians. At least for weight loss trials, characteristic findings are successful behavior change over the short term, usually 6 months or less, and then subsequent recidivism. The limited long-term success of these intensive intervention programs highlights the importance of environmental and policy changes that facilitate adoption of desirable lifestyle changes broadly across whole populations.

SPECIAL POPULATIONS
Children

The problem of elevated BP begins early in life, perhaps in utero. Numerous observational studies have documented that BP tracks from childhood into adulthood.[80] Hence, efforts to reduce BP in children and prevent the age-related rise in BP seem prudent. The importance of efforts to reduce BP in children is highlighted by evidence that BP levels and the prevalence of obesity in children and adolescents have increased between NHANES conducted in 1988 to 1994 and 1999 to 2000.[81] The relevance of sodium reduction in children is highlighted by a meta-analysis of trials in children, in which reduced dietary sodium interventions lowered BP.[82] In addition, observational studies have documented that US children have BP levels that exceed BP levels of middle-aged adults in populations exposed to a low-sodium diet.[83]

Otherwise, evidence on the effects of dietary factors on BP in children is limited and has methodological limitations, including small sample size, suboptimal BP measurements, and limited dietary contrast. Accordingly, the BP effects of diet in children and adolescents is extrapolated from studies conducted in adults. Such extrapolations are reasonable, because elevated BP is a chronic condition resulting from the insidious rise in BP throughout childhood and adulthood.

Older-Aged Persons

Dietary strategies should be especially beneficial as adults age. The age-related rise in BP is particularly prominent in middle-aged and older-aged persons, and the incidence of BP-related CV disease is especially high in older-aged persons. Although most diet-BP trials were conducted in middle-aged persons, several were conducted in older-aged individuals. Other trials have presented results stratified by age. Several important findings emerge. First, evidence is remarkably consistent that older-aged persons can make and sustain dietary changes, specifically dietary sodium reduction and weight loss.[84] Second, BP reduction from dietary interventions is greater in older-aged persons in comparison to middle-aged individuals.[23] Third, because of high attributable risk associated with elevated BP in the elderly, the beneficial effects of dietary changes on BP should reduce CV risk substantially.

African Americans

In comparison to whites, African Americans have higher BP and are at greater risk of BP-related complications, especially stroke and kidney disease. As documented previously,[23,47] in well-controlled efficacy trials, African Americans achieve greater BP reduction than whites from several nonpharmacologic therapies, specifically, sodium reduction, increased potassium intake, and the DASH diet. The potential benefits of modifying these dietary factors is amplified because survey data indicate that, on average, African Americans consume high levels of sodium whereas their potassium intake, on average, is less than that of whites.[48] In this setting, the potential benefits of dietary change are substantial and should provide a means to reduce racial disparities in BP and its CV and renal complications.[85]

Health Care Providers

A clinician's office can be a powerful setting to advocate and accomplish lifestyle change. Through advice and by example, physicians can have a substantial influence on their patients' willingness to make lifestyle changes. Although behavioral counseling is usually beyond the scope of many office practices, simple assessments and provision of advice are typically feasible (eg, calculation of BMI). The success of physician-directed, office-based attempts to achieve lifestyle changes depends on several factors, including the skills of the physician and staff, available resources, organizational structure of the office, and availability of algorithms that incorporate locally available resources. The Centers for Medicare & Medicaid Services decided to cover intensive behavioral therapy for weight-control interventions delivered in the primary care setting; however, available data are more persuasive for interventions delivered by nonphysicians in settings other than the medical office.[86]

Individualized, physician-directed efforts should be guided, in large part, by a patient's willingness to adopt lifestyle changes. Motivated patients should be referred to a skilled dietitian, health educator, or behavioral change program, because success in clinical trials has typically required frequent visits and other contacts. Even without the assistance of ancillary personnel and programs, health care providers should routinely encourage lifestyle modification.

SUMMARY

A compelling body of evidence supports the concept that multiple dietary factors affect BP. **Table 1** provides a summary of this evidence, and **Table 2** provides a summary of recommendations. Dietary changes that effectively lower BP are weight loss, reduced sodium intake, increased potassium intake, moderation of alcohol intake (among those who drink), and DASH-style and vegetarian dietary patterns. Other dietary factors may also affect BP, but the effects are small and/or the evidence uncertain.

In view of the increasing levels of BP in children and adults and the continuing epidemic of BP-related CV and renal diseases, efforts to reduce BP in both nonhypertensive and hypertensive individuals are warranted. Such efforts require

Table 1
A summary of the evidence on the effects of dietary factors and dietary patterns on blood pressure

	Hypothesized Effect	Evidence
Weight	Direct	++
Sodium chloride (salt)	Direct	++
Potassium	Inverse	++
Magnesium	Inverse	+/−
Calcium	Inverse	+/−
Alcohol	Direct	++
Fat		
Saturated fat	Direct	+/−
Omega-3 polyunsaturated fat	Inverse	++
Omega-6 polyunsaturated fat	Inverse	+/−
Monounsaturated fat	Inverse	+
Protein		
Total protein	Uncertain	+
Vegetable protein	Inverse	+
Animal protein	Uncertain	+/−
Carbohydrate	Uncertain	+/−
Fiber	Inverse	+
Cholesterol	Direct	+/−
Vitamin C	Inverse	+/−
Dietary patterns		
Vegetarian diets	Inverse	++
DASH diet	Inverse	++
Mediterranean	Inverse	+

Key to evidence: +/−, limited or equivocal evidence; +, suggestive evidence, typically from observational studies and some clinical trials; ++, persuasive evidence, typically from clinical trials.
Adapted from Appel LJ, Brands MW, Daniels SR, et al. Dietary approaches to prevent and treat hypertension: a scientific statement from the American Heart Association. Hypertension 2006;47(2):304; with permission.

individuals to change behavior and society to make environmental changes that encourage such changes. The challenge to health care providers, researchers, government officials, and the general public is developing and implementing effective clinical and public health strategies that lead to sustained dietary changes among individuals and, more broadly, among whole populations.

Table 2
Diet-related lifestyle recommendations that lower blood pressure

Lifestyle Modification	Recommendation
Weight loss	For overweight or obese persons, lose weight, ideally attaining a BMI <25 kg/m². For nonoverweight persons, maintain desirable BMI <25 kg/m².
Reduced sodium intake	Lower sodium intake as much as possible, with a goal of no more than 2300 mg/d in the general population and no more than 1500 mg/d in blacks, middle-aged and older-aged persons, and individuals with hypertension, diabetics, or CKD.
Dietary pattern	Consume a DASH-style dietary pattern rich in fruits and vegetables (8–10 servings/d), rich in low-fat dairy products (2–3 servings/d), and reduced in saturated fat and cholesterol. Vegetarian diets and to a lesser extent, Mediterranean style diets, are effective options.
Increased potassium intake	Increase potassium intake to 4.7 g/d, which is also the level provided in the DASH diet.
Moderation of alcohol intake	For those who drink alcohol, consume ≤2 alcoholic drinks/d (men) and ≤1 alcohol drink/d (women).

From Appel LJ, Brands MW, Daniels SR, et al. Dietary approaches to prevent and treat hypertension: a scientific statement from the American Heart Association. Hypertension 2006;47(2):297; with permission.

REFERENCES

1. Kearney PM, Whelton M, Reynolds K, et al. Global burden of hypertension: analysis of worldwide data. Lancet 2005;365(9455):217–23.
2. Nwankwo T, Yoon SS, Burt V, et al. Hypertension among adults in the United States: national health and nutrition examination survey, 2011-2012. NCHS Data Brief 2013;(133):1–8.
3. Whelton PK. The elusiveness of population-wide high blood pressure control. Annu Rev Public Health 2015;36:109–30.
4. Vasan RS, Beiser A, Seshadri S, et al. Residual lifetime risk for developing hypertension in middle-aged women and men: the Framingham Heart Study. JAMA 2002;287(8):1003–10.
5. Chobanian AVBG, Black HR, etal. Seventh report of the joint national committee on prevention, detection, evaluation, and treatment of high blood pressure. Hypertension 2003;(42):1206–52.
6. Lewington S, Clarke R, Qizilbash N, et al. Age-specific relevance of usual blood pressure to vascular mortality: a meta-analysis of individual data for one million adults in 61 prospective studies. Lancet 2002;360(9349):1903–13.
7. Vasan RS, Larson MG, Leip EP, et al. Impact of high-normal blood pressure on the risk of cardiovascular disease. N Engl J Med 2001;345(18):1291–7.
8. Lawes CM, Vander Hoorn S, Rodgers A. Global burden of blood-pressure-related disease, 2001. Lancet 2008;371(9623):1513–8.
9. Stamler R. Implications of the INTERSALT study. Hypertension 1991;17(1 Suppl):I16–20.
10. Sacks FM, Campos H. Dietary therapy in hypertension. N Engl J Med 2010;362(22):2102–12.
11. Appel LJ, Giles TD, Black HR, et al. ASH position paper: dietary approaches to lower blood pressure. J Am Soc Hypertens 2010;4(2):79–89.
12. Appel LJ, Brands MW, Daniels SR, et al. Dietary approaches to prevent and treat hypertension: a scientific statement from the American Heart Association. Hypertension 2006;47(2):296–308.
13. Ogden CL, Carroll MD, Kit BK, et al. Prevalence of childhood and adult obesity in the United States, 2011-2012. JAMA 2014;311(8):806–14.
14. Neter JE, Stam BE, Kok FJ, et al. Influence of weight reduction on blood pressure: a meta-analysis of randomized controlled trials. Hypertension 2003;42(5):878–84.
15. Stevens VJ, Obarzanek E, Cook NR, et al. Long-term weight loss and changes in blood pressure: results of the Trials of Hypertension Prevention, phase II. Ann Intern Med 2001;134(1):1–11.
16. Wing RR. Long-term effects of a lifestyle intervention on weight and cardiovascular risk factors in individuals with type 2 diabetes mellitus: four-year results of the Look AHEAD trial. Arch Intern Med 2010;170(17):1566–75.
17. Svetkey LP, Stevens VJ, Brantley PJ, et al. Comparison of strategies for sustaining weight loss: the weight loss maintenance randomized controlled trial. JAMA 2008;299(10):1139–48.
18. Knowler WC, Barrett-Connor E, Fowler SE, et al. Reduction in the incidence of type 2 diabetes with lifestyle intervention or metformin. N Engl J Med 2002;346(6):393–403.

19. Mozaffarian D, Fahimi S, Singh GM, et al. Global sodium consumption and death from cardiovascular causes. N Engl J Med 2014;371(7):624–34.

20. Pimenta E, Gaddam KK, Oparil S, et al. Effects of dietary sodium reduction on blood pressure in subjects with resistant hypertension: results from a randomized trial. Hypertension 2009;54(3):475–81.

21. Sacks FM, Svetkey LP, Vollmer WM, et al. Effects on blood pressure of reduced dietary sodium and the dietary approaches to Stop hypertension (DASH) diet. DASH-Sodium Collaborative Research Group. N Engl J Med 2001;344(1):3–10.

22. Johnson AG, Nguyen TV, Davis D. Blood pressure is linked to salt intake and modulated by the angiotensinogen gene in normotensive and hypertensive elderly subjects. J Hypertens 2001;19(6):1053–60.

23. Vollmer WM, Sacks FM, Ard J, et al. Effects of diet and sodium intake on blood pressure: subgroup analysis of the DASH-sodium trial. Ann Intern Med 2001;135(12):1019–28.

24. Bray GA, Vollmer WM, Sacks FM, et al. A further subgroup analysis of the effects of the DASH diet and three dietary sodium levels on blood pressure: results of the DASH-Sodium Trial. Am J Cardiol 2004;94(2):222–7.

25. Appel LJ, Espeland MA, Easter L, et al. Effects of reduced sodium intake on hypertension control in older individuals: results from the Trial of Nonpharmacologic Interventions in the Elderly (TONE). Arch Intern Med 2001;161(5):685–93.

26. Cook NR, Cutler JA, Obarzanek E, et al. Long term effects of dietary sodium reduction on cardiovascular disease outcomes: observational follow-up of the trials of hypertension prevention (TOHP). BMJ 2007; 334(7599):885–8.

27. O'Donnell M, Mente A, Rangarajan S, et al. Urinary sodium and potassium excretion, mortality, and cardiovascular events. N Engl J Med 2014;371(7):612–23.

28. Cobb LK, Anderson CA, Elliott P, et al. Methodological issues in cohort studies that relate sodium intake to cardiovascular disease outcomes: a science advisory from the American Heart Association. Circulation 2014;129(10):1173–86.

29. Chang HY, Hu YW, Yue CS, et al. Effect of potassium-enriched salt on cardiovascular mortality and medical expenses of elderly men. Am J Clin Nutr 2006;83(6):1289–96.

30. He FJ, MacGregor GA. Salt reduction lowers cardiovascular risk: meta-analysis of outcome trials. Lancet 2011;378(9789):380–2.

31. Strazzullo P, D'Elia L, Kandala NB, et al. Salt intake, stroke, and cardiovascular disease: meta-analysis of prospective studies. BMJ 2009;339:b4567.

32. Obarzanek E, Proschan MA, Vollmer WM, et al. Individual blood pressure responses to changes in salt intake: results from the DASH-Sodium trial. Hypertension 2003;42(4):459–67.

33. He FJ, Markandu ND, MacGregor GA. Importance of the renin system for determining blood pressure fall with acute salt restriction in hypertensive and normotensive whites. Hypertension 2001;38(3): 321–5.

34. Johnson RJ, Herrera-Acosta J, Schreiner GF, et al. Subtle acquired renal injury as a mechanism of salt-sensitive hypertension. N Engl J Med 2002; 346(12):913–23.

35. Frohlich ED. The salt conundrum: a hypothesis. Hypertension 2007;50(1):161–6.

36. He FJ, MacGregor GA. Effect of modest salt reduction on blood pressure: a meta-analysis of randomized trials. Implications for public health. J Hum Hypertens 2002;16(11):761–70.

37. Harsha DW, Sacks FM, Obarzanek E, et al. Effect of dietary sodium intake on blood lipids: results from the DASH-sodium trial. Hypertension 2004;43(2): 393–8.

38. Psaty BM, Lumley T, Furberg CD, et al. Health outcomes associated with various antihypertensive therapies used as first-line agents: a network meta-analysis. JAMA 2003;289(19):2534–44.

39. Centers for Disease Control and Prevention (CDC). Application of lower sodium intake recommendations to adults–United States, 1999-2006. MMWR Morb Mortal Wkly Rep 2009;58(11):281–3.

40. Lloyd-Jones DM, Hong Y, Labarthe D, et al. Defining and setting national goals for cardiovascular health promotion and disease reduction: the American Heart Association's strategic Impact Goal through 2020 and beyond. Circulation 2010;121(4):586–613.

41. Havas S, Dickinson BD, Wilson M. The urgent need to reduce sodium consumption. JAMA 2007; 298(12):1439–41.

42. Institute of Medicine (U.S.). Committee on strategies to reduce sodium intake. In: Henney JE, Taylor CL, Boon CS, editors. Strategies to reduce sodium intake in the United States. Washington, DC: National Academies Press; 2010. p. xii, 493.

43. Geleijnse JM, Kok FJ, Grobbee DE. Blood pressure response to changes in sodium and potassium intake: a metaregression analysis of randomised trials. J Hum Hypertens 2003;17(7):471–80.

44. Naismith DJ, Braschi A. The effect of low-dose potassium supplementation on blood pressure in apparently healthy volunteers. Br J Nutr 2003; 90(1):53–60.

45. Appel LJ, Moore TJ, Obarzanek E, et al. A clinical trial of the effects of dietary patterns on blood pressure. DASH Collaborative Research Group. N Engl J Med 1997;336(16):1117–24.

46. John JH, Ziebland S, Yudkin P, et al. Effects of fruit and vegetable consumption on plasma antioxidant concentrations and blood pressure: a randomised controlled trial. Lancet 2002;359(9322): 1969–74.

47. Morris RC Jr, Sebastian A, Forman A, et al. Normotensive salt sensitivity: effects of race and dietary potassium. Hypertension 1999;33(1):18–23.

48. Institute of Medicine (U.S.). Panel on dietary reference intakes for electrolytes and water. DRI, dietary reference intakes for water, potassium, sodium, chloride, and sulfate. Washington, DC: National Academies Press; 2005. p. xviii, 617.

49. K/DOQI clinical practice guidelines on hypertension and antihypertensive agents in chronic kidney disease. Am J Kidney Dis 2004;43(5 Suppl 1):S1–290.

50. Xin X, He J, Frontini MG, et al. Effects of alcohol reduction on blood pressure: a meta-analysis of randomized controlled trials. Hypertension 2001;38(5):1112–7.

51. Okubo Y, Miyamoto T, Suwazono Y, et al. Alcohol consumption and blood pressure in Japanese men. Alcohol 2001;23(3):149–56.

52. Armstrong B, van Merwyk AJ, Coates H. Blood pressure in seventh-day adventist vegetarians. Am J Epidemiol 1977;105(5):444–9.

53. Yokoyama Y, Nishimura K, Barnard ND, et al. Vegetarian diets and blood pressure: a meta-analysis. JAMA Intern Med 2014;174(4):577–87.

54. Appel LJ, Sacks FM, Carey VJ, et al. Effects of protein, monounsaturated fat, and carbohydrate intake on blood pressure and serum lipids: results of the OmniHeart randomized trial. JAMA 2005;294(19):2455–64.

55. Sofi F, Abbate R, Gensini GF, et al. Accruing evidence on benefits of adherence to the Mediterranean diet on health: an updated systematic review and meta-analysis. Am J Clin Nutr 2010;92(5):1189–96.

56. Estruch R, Ros E, Salas-Salvado J, et al. Primary prevention of cardiovascular disease with a Mediterranean diet. N Engl J Med 2013;368(14):1279–90.

57. Nordmann AJ, Suter-Zimmermann K, Bucher HC, et al. Meta-analysis comparing Mediterranean to low-fat diets for modification of cardiovascular risk factors. Am J Med 2011;124(9):841–51.e2.

58. Campbell F, Dickinson HO, Critchley JA, et al. A systematic review of fish-oil supplements for the prevention and treatment of hypertension. Eur J Prev Cardiol 2013;20(1):107–20.

59. Streppel MT, Arends LR, van 't Veer P, et al. Dietary fiber and blood pressure: a meta-analysis of randomized placebo-controlled trials. Arch Intern Med 2005;165(2):150–6.

60. Whelton SP, Hyre AD, Pedersen B, et al. Effect of dietary fiber intake on blood pressure: a meta-analysis of randomized, controlled clinical trials. J Hypertens 2005;23(3):475–81.

61. Cappuccio FP, Elliott P, Allender PS, et al. Epidemiologic association between dietary calcium intake and blood pressure: a meta-analysis of published data. Am J Epidemiol 1995;142(9):935–45.

62. Allender PS, Cutler JA, Follmann D, et al. Dietary calcium and blood pressure: a meta-analysis of randomized clinical trials. Ann Intern Med 1996;124(9):825–31.

63. Jee SH, Miller ER 3rd, Guallar E, et al. The effect of magnesium supplementation on blood pressure: a meta-analysis of randomized clinical trials. Am J Hypertens 2002;15(8):691–6.

64. Ferrara LA, Raimondi AS, d'Episcopo L, et al. Olive oil and reduced need for antihypertensive medications. Arch Intern Med 2000;160(6):837–42.

65. Shah M, Adams-Huet B, Garg A. Effect of high-carbohydrate or high-cis-monounsaturated fat diets on blood pressure: a meta-analysis of intervention trials. Am J Clin Nutr 2007;85(5):1251–6.

66. Sacks FM, Carey VJ, Anderson CA, et al. Effects of high vs low glycemic index of dietary carbohydrate on cardiovascular disease risk factors and insulin sensitivity: the OmniCarb randomized clinical trial. JAMA 2014;312(23):2531–41.

67. Dhingra R, Sullivan L, Jacques PF, et al. Soft drink consumption and risk of developing cardiometabolic risk factors and the metabolic syndrome in middle-aged adults in the community. Circulation 2007;116(5):480–8.

68. Chen L, Caballero B, Mitchell DC, et al. Reducing consumption of sugar-sweetened beverages is associated with reduced blood pressure: a prospective study among United States adults. Circulation 2010;121(22):2398–406.

69. Visvanathan R, Chen R, Horowitz M, et al. Blood pressure responses in healthy older people to 50 g carbohydrate drinks with differing glycaemic effects. Br J Nutr 2004;92(2):335–40.

70. Stamler J, Liu K, Ruth KJ, et al. Eight-year blood pressure change in middle-aged men: relationship to multiple nutrients. Hypertension 2002;39(5):1000–6.

71. Elliott P, Stamler J, Dyer AR, et al. Association between protein intake and blood pressure: the INTERMAP Study. Arch Intern Med 2006;166(1):79–87.

72. Rebholz CM, Friedman EE, Powers LJ, et al. Dietary protein intake and blood pressure: a meta-analysis of randomized controlled trials. Am J Epidemiol 2012;176(Suppl 7):S27–43.

73. Juraschek SP, Guallar E, Appel LJ, et al. Effects of vitamin C supplementation on blood pressure: a meta-analysis of randomized controlled trials. Am J Clin Nutr 2012;95(5):1079–88.

74. Lifton RP, Wilson FH, Choate KA, et al. Salt and blood pressure: new insight from human genetic studies. Cold Spring Harb Symp Quant Biol 2002;67:445–50.

75. Svetkey LP, Moore TJ, Simons-Morton DG, et al. Angiotensinogen genotype and blood pressure response in the Dietary Approaches to Stop Hypertension (DASH) study. J Hypertens 2001;19(11):1949–56.

76. Grant FD, Romero JR, Jeunemaitre X, et al. Low-renin hypertension, altered sodium homeostasis, and an alpha-adducin polymorphism. Hypertension 2002;39(2):191–6.

77. Kostis JB, Wilson AC, Hooper WC, et al. Association of angiotensin-converting enzyme DD genotype with blood pressure sensitivity to weight loss. Am Heart J 2002;144(4):625–9.

78. Miller ER 3rd, Erlinger TP, Young DR, et al. Results of the diet, exercise, and weight loss intervention trial (DEW-IT). Hypertension 2002;40(5):612–8.

79. Appel LJ, Champagne CM, Harsha DW, et al. Effects of comprehensive lifestyle modification on blood pressure control: main results of the PREMIER clinical trial. JAMA 2003;289(16):2083–93.

80. Dekkers JC, Snieder H, Van Den Oord EJ, et al. Moderators of blood pressure development from childhood to adulthood: a 10-year longitudinal study. J Pediatr 2002;141(6):770–9.

81. Muntner P, He J, Cutler JA, et al. Trends in blood pressure among children and adolescents. JAMA 2004;291(17):2107–13.

82. He FJ, MacGregor GA. Importance of salt in determining blood pressure in children: meta-analysis of controlled trials. Hypertension 2006;48(5):861–9.

83. Appel LJ. At the tipping point: accomplishing population-wide sodium reduction in the United States. J Clin Hypertens (Greenwich) 2008;10(1):7–11.

84. Whelton PK, Appel LJ, Espeland MA, et al. Sodium reduction and weight loss in the treatment of hypertension in older persons: a randomized controlled trial of nonpharmacologic interventions in the elderly (TONE). TONE Collaborative Research Group. JAMA 1998;279(11):839–46.

85. Erlinger TP, Vollmer WM, Svetkey LP, et al. The potential impact of nonpharmacologic population-wide blood pressure reduction on coronary heart disease events: pronounced benefits in African-Americans and hypertensives. Prev Med 2003; 37(4):327–33.

86. Wadden TA, Butryn ML, Hong PS, et al. Behavioral treatment of obesity in patients encountered in primary care settings: a systematic review. JAMA 2014;312(17):1779–91.

The Environment and Blood Pressure

Robert D. Brook, MD

KEYWORDS

• Air pollution • Temperature • Altitude • Noise • Hypertension • Cardiovascular risk

KEY POINTS

• Numerous environmental factors including cold weather, winter season, higher altitude, loud noises, and air pollutants can acutely increase blood pressure.
• Long-term exposures to many of these environmental factors may promote the development of chronic hypertension.
• Health care providers should be aware of these associations and take practical steps to monitor blood pressure closely during exposures to avoid worsening of hypertension.

Hypertension most often arises as a consequence of adverse lifestyle environmental factors (eg, high sodium intake, obesity) in the setting of an underlying polygenetic predisposition.[1] In modern-day societies it is a burgeoning public health epidemic whereby high blood pressure (BP) now accounts for nearly half of all cardiovascular events and is the leading risk factor for morbidity and mortality worldwide.[1,2] Fortunately, many medications and behavioral interventions (eg, reduced sodium intake, weight loss) have proven to lower BP and reduce cardiovascular risk in numerous clinical trials.[1] On the other hand, far less attention in clinical practice has been paid to the importance of several additional environmental factors also associated with high BP.[3] Mounting evidence shows that colder outdoor temperatures, winter season, higher altitudes, loud noises, and ambient air pollutants are each capable of elevating BP.[3] Although the individual BP-raising effects are generally modest (5–15 mm Hg), billions of people are affected daily given their omnipresent nature. Hence, the adverse impacts on overall BP control and cardiovascular risk at the global public health level are likely substantial. This review discusses the evidence linking exposures to several environmental factors with high

BP and briefly outlines the potential implications for clinical practice.[3]

COLD AMBIENT TEMPERATURE AND WINTER SEASON

Colder outdoor temperature levels increase BP over a few hours to days (**Table 1**).[3–13] A wide range of studies across many populations and climates has consistently reported an inverse association between BP and ambient temperature during the preceding few days.[3–10,14–24] In a large study of more than 500,000 people across China, a 10°C colder temperature was associated with a 5.7-mm Hg increase in systolic BP.[14] Compared with summer, systolic BP was approximately 10 mm Hg higher during winter seasons. In Michigan, similar associations were observed among 2078 cardiac rehabilitation patients. A reduction in outdoor temperature levels by 10.4°C during the prior 1 to 7 days promoted a 3.6-mm Hg increase in systolic BP.[21] Several additional recent studies are notable for reporting similar findings including in patients with cardiovascular disease,[15] individuals residing in rural China (eg, 13% lower hypertension control rate during winter),[16] and in Dutch (n = 101,377)[18] and Italian populations.[19,20]

Disclosures: The author has nothing to disclose.
Division of Cardiovascular Medicine, University of Michigan, 24 Frank Lloyd Wright Drive, PO Box 322, Ann Arbor, MI 48188, USA
E-mail address: robdbrok@umich.edu

Cardiol Clin 35 (2017) 213–221
http://dx.doi.org/10.1016/j.ccl.2016.12.003
0733-8651/17/© 2016 Elsevier Inc. All rights reserved.

Table 1
Environmental exposures and blood pressure

	Exposure Effect on Blood Pressure	Possible Mechanism(s)
Temperature	Overall: Inverse association	Thermoregulation-mediated vasoconstriction
Cold	Colder ambient temperature increases BP	HPAA and SNS activation, sodium retention Impaired endothelial-dependent vasodilatation
Heat	Warmer daytime associated with higher nocturnal BP	Possibly reduced sleep quality
Season	Overall: Winter associated with higher BP	Cold-induced mechanisms (above)
Winter	BP may be 5–10 mm Hg higher during winter.	Possible additional alterations may play roles: lower vitamin D, reduced activity, weight gain, shifts in fluid balance (aldosterone increase), and increased arterial stiffness
Geography	Overall: Higher altitude (>2500 m) raises BP	Altitude-induced hypoxemia activates the chemoreflex causing increased SNS and adrenal activity. Long-term acclimatization may lead to differing responses.
Altitude	Magnitude of effect may be impacted by race, acclimatization and rate of ascent, as well as duration of exposure.	Other factors such as cold and stress may also play a role. Long-term increases in red blood cell mass may contribute
Loud noises	Overall: Exposure to loud noises raises BP. Living near loud noise conditions (traffic) promotes chronic hypertension Numerous conditions implicated (traffic, airports)	Acute SNS activation, HPAA activation, endothelial dysfunction Possibly impaired sleep quality
Pollutants	Overall: Exposure to air pollutants raises BP	Acute activation of the SNS, systemic inflammation, or constituents reaching the systemic vasculature and promoting vasoconstriction
Ambient PM	Short and long-term PM exposures related to higher BP and increased hypertension onset	
Indoor PM	Multiple size ranges (fine, coarse, ultrafine) of PM and sources (urban, rural, biomass, and personal-level) of exposures implicated	Chronic exposures likely alter vascular tone via endothelial dysfunction or reduced arterial compliance due to PM-mediated inflammation and oxidative stress in the vasculature and in the central nervous system.
SHS	SHS exposure increases BP	
Other Exposures	Metals (lead, cadmium, arsenic, mercury), POP, bisphenol A strong odors, phthalates	Unclear

Abbreviations: PM, particulate matter; POP, persistent organic pollutants.

BP levels are often highest during winter months.[14] Some findings support that this chronic seasonal variation occurs above and beyond the acute impact of cold ambient temperature levels during the prior few days.[14,16,19] Moreover, an opposite hemodynamic effect of nocturnal ambient temperatures has been illustrated. Nighttime BP is found to be higher during summer (ie, warmer days) compared with winter months.[7,10,19,20] There are also potential differential effects of indoor versus outdoor temperature exposures and important considerations with regard to the possible mitigating actions of household heating during winter months.[10,14,19] Taken together, the existing studies show that on average, colder temperatures and winter months are associated with higher BP levels. However, there are additional complex interrelationships involving several exposure parameters (time of day, durations, indoor vs outdoor temperatures) that determine the full nature of the physiologic responses.

Several mechanisms are likely responsible for the BP-raising effects of cold. Acute exposure principally increases BP via arteriolar vasoconstriction as part of the thermo-regulatory response.[8] Hypothalamic pituitary adrenal axis (HPAA) and sympathetic nervous system (SNS) activation are also involved (see **Table 1**). Additional physiologic adaptations (eg, lower Vitamin D, weight gain, reduced activity, and changes in diet/fluid balance) likely play further mechanistic roles in the more chronic seasonal effects.

Both colder ambient temperatures and winter seasons can produce clinically meaningful elevations in BP and may possibly play an important role in the increase in cardiovascular events known to occur during winter.[25,26] Some evidence supports that hypertensive patients should monitor their BP particularly closely during colder weather and throughout the winter.[14,16,27] A substantial number of patients (38% in one study)[28] may require adjustments or additions to their antihypertensive regimens to maintain BP control. Although epidemiologic studies suggest that residential heating might mitigate the prohypertensive effects of cold,[11,14] further studies are needed in this regard. The effectiveness of other practical personal-level lifestyle actions (eg, using space heaters, wearing warmer clothes, avoiding outdoor cold temperatures) that individuals with hypertension can take to lessen the ill effects of cold remains unclear and requires further investigation before making any clinical recommendations.

LOUD NOISES

A large array of loud noises has been implicated in increasing BP, including those from urban (eg, traffic, airplanes) and occupational (eg, machinery) sources (see **Table 1**).[29–36] Similar to cold temperatures, brief exposures are capable of increasing BP within minutes.[31,32] Mounting evidence further supports that residing in locations chronically impacted by loud noise (eg, nearby traffic and airports) increases the risk for overt hypertension over the long term.[29,30,33] Whether specific sources are more or less harmful remains to be clarified; however, some studies suggest that nighttime exposures to loud noises (ie, from aircraft noise) have a particularly detrimental impact on increasing BP.[32]

Several recent studies have provided yet further evidence of the adverse short- and long-term effects of noise on BP.[35] The best available overall estimate of the chronic impact comes from a meta-analysis of 24 cross-sectional studies, which found a 7% increase in the prevalence of hypertension per 10 dB increase in estimated 16-hour average traffic noise exposure.[36] Residing near roadways has also been associated with high BP. In a large cohort (>38,000) of women across the United States, a household residence within 50 m of a major roadway was independently linked to a 13% higher incidence of hypertension.[37] Given that several different environmental exposures may be involved in the BP-raising effects of living near roads, several studies have attempted to dissociate the ill effects of noise from other coexposures (eg, air pollution). An individual contribution of noise on promoting high BP has been supported in some[38,39] but not all studies.[40]

Several germane physiologic pathways, whereby loud noises can mediate an acute increase in BP and promote the chronic development of hypertension, have been described (see **Table 1**).[35] Important mechanisms seem to be heightened sympathetic nervous system activity, an increase in circulating stress hormones, and activation of the hypothalamic pituitary adrenal axis. Nighttime exposure seems capable of disrupting sleep quality and vascular endothelial function, even when an individual is not awoken by the noise.[35,41,42]

The global health importance of excessive noise continues to grow. Recent estimates are that half the world's population now lives in cities,[37] and roughly 40% of Europeans face excess traffic noise.[35] Perhaps 150 million people living in the United States are exposed to noise levels, placing them at increased risk for hypertension.[43] It is plausible that the BP-raising effect of loud noise plays a key role in at least partially explaining the growing number of studies reporting associations between traffic[44,45] or aircraft[46,47] noise and increased cardiovascular events. Although urban planning and local noise ordinances can lessen exposures,[43,48] the steps that individual patients can take to reduce the harmful impacts of noise are less clearly defined. One obvious prudent action is to avoid intense noise exposures when possible, particularly among high-risk hypertensive and coronary disease patients. The effectiveness of using personal protection devices at work (eg, ear muffs), home (eg, close windows, use noise silencers), or during hospitalization to reduce exposures and prevent increases in BP requires furthers study. Finally, the maximal noise intensity threshold that is safe with regard to BP and cardiovascular risk remains to be clarified.

HIGHER ALTITUDES

Ascent to higher altitudes increases BP (see **Table 1**). The BP-raising effects can occur over a few days and are independent of the often concomitant exposure to colder temperatures.[49–54] However, the absolute magnitude of hemodynamic changes varies substantially among individuals and may even differ between races.[49,51] The acuity of ascent also appears to be important, as those who have acclimatized over weeks often exhibit smaller elevations in BP.[51] Few studies have evaluated the long-term impact; however, recent studies suggest that the pressor response may persist for weeks to months when remaining at a higher altitude.[50,55,56] The altitude required to pose a threat also remains to be fully clarified. Nevertheless, the overall evidence supports that short-term ascent to above 2500 m usually elicits an increase in BP,[49–51] whereas several studies also suggest that even lower altitudes (1200 m) can also present some risk.[51]

A variety of mechanisms may be responsible. The most import biological pathway responsible is likely hypoxia-induced (because of the lower partial pressure of oxygen at higher altitude) activation of the chemoreflex at the level of the carotid body and an ensuing augmentation of sympathetic outflow (see **Table 1**).[51,54,55,57,58] Other possible physiologic pathways reported in some studies include increased arterial stiffness, endothelin release, and heightened overall blood viscosity.[51,52]

On the other hand, the evidence that living at higher altitudes promotes the development of chronic hypertension is more mixed.[53–55,59] Difficulties in studying this effect reflect the presence of multiple confounding factors such coexposures (eg, cold) and differences in other ecological, genetic, and lifestyle variables between populations living at various altitudes.[59] A recent meta-analysis of 8 studies in Tibet (n = 16,913) has helped to clarify this issue. Among individuals living at 3000 to 4300 m above sea level, there was a positive association between hypertension and higher altitude whereby a 100-m increase in altitude was independently associated with a 2% increase in hypertension prevalence.[56] These findings suggest that provided that all other important factors remain similar, living at a higher altitude may play a role in promoting chronic elevations in BP.

A few medication interventions have been evaluated in an effort to mitigate the BP-raising effects

of high altitude.[57,58] In a recent study, 24-hour BP levels were elevated among 45 participants traveling to Mt. Everest base camp.[57] There was a progressive increase in systolic BP (10–15 mm Hg) and plasma norepinephrine concentrations ascending from 3400 m up to 5400 m. These responses started immediately and persisted throughout the timeframe at high altitude. Treatment with an angiotensin receptor blockade (ARB) was not capable of mitigating the pressor response (ie, magnitude of BP elevations), whereas it did slightly lower the actual absolute BP levels (4 mm Hg) compared with placebo at 3400 m but not at higher altitudes (5400 m). This lack of efficacy is consistent with the fact that circulating markers of renin-angiotensin activity were suppressed at the higher altitudes. The investigators reported similar findings in a study of 89 patients with mild hypertension climbing 3260 m in the Andes.[58] Combination ARB plus calcium channel blocker therapy did not prove capable of blunting the magnitude of high altitude–induced BP elevations (10–15 mm Hg systolic). However, absolute BP levels remained significantly lower during combination therapy compared with placebo at all altitudes.

Guidelines for managing high BP and reducing the cardiovascular risk of patients who plan to ascend to higher altitudes (>2500 m) have been published.[52,54,60] This public health concern is not trivial given the roughly 35 million people per year travel worldwide above this altitude.[55] Current recommendations based on expert opinions involve proper acclimatization along with more scrupulous monitoring of BP during the time spent at higher altitudes.[54,60] From a clinical practice perspective, this may involve education of patients as a precaution to carefully monitor their BP during travel, vacation, or seasonal relocation to higher altitudes (perhaps even at only 1200 m above sea level among at-risk patients).[57,58] Beta blockers and ARBs do not seem to prevent the BP-raising response. However, ARB plus calcium channel blocker therapy may provide some partial protection by lowering the absolute level of BP so that the pressor response does not reduce overall BP control.[57,58] The optimal medication regimen and management strategies (eg, increase or add medications, descent to lower levels) to control altitude-induced BP elevations remains to be fully clarified.[52]

AIR POLLUTANTS

Fine particulate matter less than 2.5 μm air pollution ($PM_{2.5}$), most commonly derived from fossil fuel combustion during modern-day activities (eg, traffic, power generation, industry), is a leading risk factor for cardiovascular morbidity and mortality.[61–63] One important mechanism may be $PM_{2.5}$-induced elevations in BP (see **Table 1**). Numerous studies from across the globe[61–66] and a recent meta-analysis (up to 25 studies) found that acute exposures are capable of increasing BP (typically by 1 to 2 mm Hg per 10 $\mu g/m^3$) over a period of a few hours to days. The authors found that among 2078 heart disease patients living in southeast Michigan, typical day-to-day variations (8.2 $\mu g/m^3$) of ambient $PM_{2.5}$ during the prior few days were independently associated with significant increases in BP by 2.1 to 3.5/1.7 to 1.8 mm Hg.[21] This finding occurred despite the fact that mean $PM_{2.5}$ levels (12.6 $\mu g/m^3$) were on average within daily United States National Ambient Air Quality Standards (<35 $\mu g/m^3$).[63] Extreme $PM_{2.5}$ elevations (ranging from 50 to 750 $\mu g/m^3$), as occurs in China, have also been associated with both short-term and long-term increases in BP.[64,65] However, the impact of more chronic exposures over years is less well studied. A meta-analysis of fewer studies suggests that the BP-raising effect may be even more robust (7.3/9.5 mm Hg per 10 $\mu g/m^3$).[66] To provide experimental support for these associations, we and others have conducted several randomized, double-blind, controlled exposures to $PM_{2.5}$, coarse particulate matter (2.5–10 μm), and diesel exhaust particles (10–100 nm). Acute inhalation of particulate air pollutants across a wide range of size fractions and derived from a variety of sources were all found to be capable of increasing BP (2–10 mm Hg) within a few hours.[62]

From a real-world perspective, it is equally important to understand what the long-term health ramifications are of living over many years in locations with higher air pollution levels. Recent evidence supports that exposure to $PM_{2.5}$ on a chronic basis promotes the development of overt hypertension.[62] This occurs even in a relatively clean environment from a global perspective. Among 33,303 adults living in Ontario, Canada, an increase of $PM_{2.5}$ levels by 10 $\mu g/m^3$ was associated with a 13% higher incidence of hypertension over 14 years of follow-up.[67] A similar increase in the risk was found in association with chronic traffic-related pollution exposure among black women living in Los Angeles.[68] Recent evidence also supports that living in regions across the United States facing higher $PM_{2.5}$ levels leads to an increase in hypertension-related mortality over the long term.[69]

Numerous biological pathways were found in experimental studies to explain the mechanisms involved in air pollution–mediated BP elevations.[62,63] The inhalation of $PM_{2.5}$ interacts with a host of pulmonary receptors (transient receptor potential channels) and nerve endings (c-fibers) to initiate nervous system reflex arcs. This interaction results in an imbalance in systemic autonomic outflow favoring sympathetic tone. At the same time, the deposition of fine particles in lung airways creates a nidus of pulmonary inflammation. Local mediators including cytokines, active cells, and oxidized biological molecules (eg, phospholipids) spill over into the systemic circulation and thereafter adversely affect the function of the cardiovascular system. Finally, some pro-oxidative constituents of inhaled particles (eg, nanoparticles, metals, organic compounds) may even be capable of translocating directly into the systemic circulation and mediate direct adverse actions. Together, these responses likely elicit the arterial vasoconstriction and endothelial dysfunction, which are ultimately responsible for the increase in BP shown to occur after $PM_{2.5}$ exposure.[63]

Finally, other sources of air pollution, such as secondhand smoke (SHS) from cigarettes, can also increase BP.[70–75] Increasing evidence supports that SHS increases the risk of elevated home BP readings and for masked hypertension.[72–74] Controlled exposures[70] and personal monitoring[71] studies further suggest that short-term SHS inhalation causes elevations in BP. Mounting evidence shows that long-term exposures to SHS are also capable of promoting the development of chronic hypertension.[76,77]

The adverse effects of $PM_{2.5}$ on increasing arterial BP are clinically relevant. Studies found that emergency department visits specifically for hypertension increase after more air-polluted days.[62,78] Increased death rates over the long term caused by hypertension-related diseases are also linked to chronic $PM_{2.5}$ exposures.[69] Fortunately, national ambient air quality regulations have proven capable of producing substantial reductions in air pollution levels over the last few decades. Cardiovascular health is found to improve as a direct consequence of the improved air quality.[79] Several personal-level interventions may also reduce the harmful actions of $PM_{2.5}$ exposures include wearing facemasks while outdoors or closing outside windows while in extremely polluted cities and using in-home and automobile cabin high-efficiency particulate arrestance (HEPA) filtration systems.[79] Decreased SHS also results in reductions (10%–20%) in cardiovascular events within a few months of public smoking ordinances.[80] Clinical recommendations to assess and reduce the cardiovascular risks of air pollution have been outlined in detail previously.[63]

OTHER ENVIRONMENTAL FACTORS

A large variety of other environmental factors are also associated with higher BP levels (see **Table 1**). These factors include persistent organic pollutants, strong odors (eg, nearby farms), metals (ie, lead, cadmium, mercury, arsenic), and chemicals used in plastics (eg, bisphenol A) and food wraps (eg, phthalates).[3,81–86] Facial immersion in cold water (diving reflex) increases BP,[3] and living at more extreme northern or southern latitudes is also associated with higher BP.[81,82]

CLINICAL IMPLICATIONS

The overall burden of evidence supports that many environmental exposures have the capacity to rapidly increase BP and thereby disrupt BP control. This suggests that clinicians and individuals with hypertension should be aware of these factors and pay closer attention to BP levels during such exposures. It is possible that antihypertensive treatments and medications may need to be adjusted to maintain BP control. Other practical recommendations for health care providers include providing counseling to patients regarding the risks during activities (eg, travel, residential, or occupational moves) to environmental settings in which increased exposures are expected (eg, high altitude, colder or polluted locations). In rare circumstances it may be prudent for some very high-risk patients (eg, severely uncontrolled hypertension) to avoid unnecessary exposures if possible (eg, cancel voluntary travel). Completely avoiding exposures may be nearly impossible or require impractical life changes. On the other hand, evidence from studies is beginning to show that a few practical interventions such as avoiding SHS exposures, using in-home air purifiers with HEPA filters to reduce indoor air pollution, and keeping household residences well heated during winter months can prevent BP elevations. Further studies are urgently needed to determine practical and effective personal-level interventions that can help mitigate the adverse BP and cardiovascular health impacts of environmental exposures given their global public health ramifications.

REFERENCES

1. Mancia G, Fagard R, Narkiewicz K, et al. 2013 ESH/ESC Guidelines for the management of arterial hypertension: the Task Force for the management of arterial hypertension of the European Society of Hypertension (ESH) and of the European Society of Cardiology (ESC). J Hypertens 2013;31:1281–357.

2. GBD 2013 Risk Factors Collaborators. Global, regional, and national comparative risk assessment of 79 behavioral, environmental and occupational, and metabolic risks or clusters of risks in 188 countries, 1990-2013: a systematic analysis for the Global Burden of Disease Study 2013. Lancet 2015;386:2287–323.

3. Brook RD, Weder AB, Rajagopalan S. "Environmental hypertensionology" the effects of environmental factors on blood pressure in clinical practice and research. J Clin Hypertens (Greenwich) 2011;13:836–42.

4. Alpérovitch A, Lacombe J-M, Hanon O, et al. Relationship between blood pressure and outdoor temperature in a large sample of elderly individuals. The Three-City Study. Arch Intern Med 2009;169:75–80.

5. Barnett AG, Sans S, Salomaa V, et al. The effect of temperature on systolic blood pressure. Blood Press Monit 2007;12:195–203.

6. Halonen JI, Zanobetti A, Sparrow D, et al. Relationship between outdoor temperature and blood pressure. Occup Environ Med 2011;68:296–301.

7. Modesti PA, Borabito M, Bertolozzi I, et al. Weather-related changes in 24-hour blood pressure profile. Effects of age and implications for hypertension management. Hypertension 2006;47:1–7.

8. Sun Z. Cardiovascular responses to cold exposure. Front Biosci 2010;2:495–503.

9. Luurila AJ, Kohvakka A, Sundberg S. Comparison of blood pressure response to heat stress in sauna in young hypertensive patients treated with atenolol and diltiazem. Am J Cardiol 1989;64:97–9.

10. Brook RD, Shin HH, Bard RL, et al. Can personal exposures to higher nighttime and early morning temperatures increase blood pressure? J Clin Hypertens 2011;13(12):881–8.

11. Nafstad MC. Associations between environmental exposure and blood pressure among participants in the Oslo Health Study (HUBRO). Eur J Epidemiol 2006;21:485–91.

12. Woodhouse PR, Khaw K-T, Plummer M. Seasonal variation of blood pressure and its relationship to ambient temperature in an elderly population. J Hypertens 1993;11:1267–74.

13. Al-Tamre YY, Al-Hayali JMT, Al-Ramadhan EAH. Seasonality of hypertension. J Clin Hypertens 2008;10:125–9.

14. Lewington S, Li L, Sherliker P, et al. China Kadoorie Biobank study collaboration. Seasonal variation in blood pressure and its relationship with outdoor temperature in 10 diverse regions of China: the China Kadoorie Biobank. J Hypertens 2012;30:1383–91.

15. Yang L, Li L, Lewington S, et al. China Kadoorie Biobank Study Collaboration. Outdoor temperature, blood pressure, and cardiovascular disease mortality among 23 000 individuals with diagnosed

cardiovascular diseases from China. Eur Heart J 2015;36:1178–85.

16. Su D, Du H, Zhang X, et al. Season and outdoor temperature in relation to detection and control of hypertension in a large rural Chinese population. Int J Epidemiol 2014;43:1835–45.

17. Chen Q, Wang J, Tian J, et al. Association between ambient temperature and blood pressure and blood pressure regulators: 1831 hypertensive patients followed up for three years. PLoS One 2013;8:e84522.

18. van den Hurk K, de Kort WL, Deinum J, et al. Higher outdoor temperatures are progressively associated with lower blood pressure: a longitudinal study in 100,000 healthy individuals. J Am Soc Hypertens 2015;9:536–43.

19. Modesti PA, Morabito M, Massetti L, et al. Seasonal blood pressure changes: an independent relationship with temperature and daylight hours. Hypertension 2013;61:908–14.

20. Fedecostante M, Barbatelli P, Guerra F, et al. Summer does not always mean lower: seasonality of 24 h, daytime, and night-time blood pressure. J Hypertens 2012;30:1392–8.

21. Giorgini P, Rubenfire M, Das R, et al. Particulate matter air pollution and ambient temperature: opposing effects on blood pressure in high-risk cardiac patients. J Hypertens 2015;33:2032–8.

22. Auda F. Winter hypertension: potential mechanisms. Int J Health Sci (Qassim) 2013;7:210–9.

23. Cuspidi C, Ochoa JE, Parati G. Seasonal variations in blood pressure: a complex phenomenon. J Hypertens 2012;30:1315–20.

24. Cui J, Muller MD, Blaha C, et al. Seasonal variation in muscle sympathetic nerve activity. Physiol Rep 2015;3:e12492.

25. Ye X, Wolff R, Yu W, et al. Ambient temperature and morbidity: a review of epidemiological evidence. Environ Health Perspect 2012;120:19–28.

26. Bhaskaran K, Hajat S, Haines A, et al. Short term effects of temperature on risk of myocardial infarction in England and Wales: time series regression analysis of the Myocardial Ischaemia National Audit Project (MINAP) registry. BMJ 2010;341:c3823.

27. Handler J. Seasonal variability of blood pressure in California. J Clin Hypertens (Greenwich) 2011;13:856–60.

28. Charach G, Rabinovich PD, Weintraub M. Seasonal changes in blood pressure and frequency of related complications in elderly Israeli patients with essential hypertension. Gerontology 2004;50:315–21.

29. Jarup L, Babisch W, Houthuijs D, et al. Hypertension and exposure to noise near airports: the HYENA study. Environ Health Perspect 2008;116:329–33.

30. Barregard L, Bonde E, Öhrström E. Risk of hypertension from exposure to road traffic noise in a population-based sample. Occup Environ Med 2009;66:410–5.

31. Chang T-Y, Lai Y-A, Hsieh H-H, et al. Effects of environmental noise exposure on ambulatory blood pressure in young adults. Environ Res 2009;109:900–5.

32. Haraladbidis AS, Dimakopoulou K, Vigna-Taglianti F, et al. Acute effects of night-time noise exposure on blood pressure in populations living near airports. Eur Heart J 2008;29:658–64.

33. Davies HW, Vlaanderen JJ, Henderson SB, et al. Correlation between co-exposures to noise and air pollution from traffic sources. Occup Environ Med 2009;66:347–50.

34. Barregard L. Traffic noise and hypertension. Environ Res 2011;111:186–7.

35. Münzel T, Gori T, Babisch W, et al. Cardiovascular effects of environmental noise exposure. Eur Heart J 2014;35:829–36.

36. van Kempen E, Babisch W. The quantitative relationship between road traffic noise and hypertension: a meta-analysis. J Hypertens 2012;30:1075–86.

37. Kingsley SL, Eliot MN, Whitsel EA, et al. Residential proximity to major roadways and incident hypertension in post-menopausal women. Environ Res 2015;142:522–8.

38. Foraster M, Künzli N, Aguilera I, et al. High blood pressure and long-term exposure to indoor noise and air pollution from road traffic. Environ Health Perspect 2014;122:1193–200.

39. Stansfeld SA. Noise effects on health in the context of air pollution exposure. Int J Environ Res Public Health 2015;12:12735–60.

40. Babisch W, Wolf K, Petz M, et al. Associations between traffic noise, particulate air pollution, hypertension, and isolated systolic hypertension in adults: the KORA study. Environ Health Perspect 2014;122:492–8.

41. Akinseye OA, Williams SK, Seixas A, et al. Sleep as a mediator in the pathway linking environmental factors to hypertension: a review of the literature. Int J Hypertens 2015;2015:926414.

42. Schmidt F, Kolle K, Kreuder K, et al. Nighttime aircraft noise impairs endothelial function and increases blood pressure in patients with or at high risk for coronary artery disease. Clin Res Cardiol 2015;104:23–30.

43. Hammer MS, Swinburn TK, Neitzel RL. Environmental noise pollution in the United States: developing an effective public health response. Environ Health Perspect 2014;122:115–9.

44. Babisch W. Updated exposure-response relationship between road traffic noise and coronary heart diseases: a meta-analysis. Noise Health 2014;16:1–9.

45. Halonen JI, Hansell AL, Gulliver J, et al. Road traffic noise is associated with increased cardiovascular morbidity and mortality and all-cause mortality in London. Eur Heart J 2015;36:2653–61.

46. Floud S, Blangiardo M, Clark C, et al. Exposure to aircraft and road traffic noise and associations with heart disease and stroke in six European countries: a cross-sectional study. Environ Health 2013;12:89.

47. Correia AW, Peters JL, Levy JI, et al. Residential exposure to aircraft noise and hospital admissions for cardiovascular diseases: multi-airport retrospective study. BMJ 2013;347:f5561.

48. Babisch W, Swart W, Houthuijs D, et al. Exposure modifiers of the relationships of transportation noise with high blood pressure and noise annoyance. J Acoust Soc Am 2012;132:3788–808.

49. Hasler E, Suter PM, Vetter W. Race specific altitude effects on blood pressure. J Hum Hypertens 1997; 11(7):435–8.

50. Sizlan A, Ogur R, Ozer M, et al. Blood pressure changes in young male subjects exposed to a median altitude. Clin Auton Res 2008;18:84–9.

51. Handler J. Altitude-related hypertension. J Clin Hypertens 2009;11:161–5.

52. Luks AM. Should travelers with hypertension adjust their medications when traveling to high altitude? High Alt Med Biol 2009;10:11–4.

53. Faeh D, Gutzwiller F, Bopp M, et al. Lower mortality from coronary heart disease and stroke at higher altitudes in Switzerland. Circulation 2009;120: 495–501.

54. Rimoldi SF, Sartori C, Seiler C, et al. High-altitude exposure in patients with cardiovascular disease: risk assessment and practical recommendations. Prog Cardiovasc Dis 2010;52:512–24.

55. Dhar P, Sharma VK, Hota KB, et al. Autonomic cardiovascular responses in acclimatized lowlanders on prolonged stay at high altitude: a longitudinal follow up study. PLoS One 2014;9:e84274.

56. Mingji C, Onakpoya IJ, Perera R, et al. Relationship between altitude and the prevalence of hypertension in Tibet: a systematic review. Heart 2015;101: 1054–60.

57. Parati G, Bilo G, Faini A, et al. Changes in 24 h ambulatory blood pressure and effects of angiotensin II receptor blockade during acute and prolonged high-altitude exposure: a randomized clinical trial. Eur Heart J 2014;35:3113–22.

58. Bilo G, Villafuerte FC, Faini A, et al. Ambulatory blood pressure in untreated and treated hypertensive patients at high altitude: the high altitude cardiovascular research-andes study. Hypertension 2015;65:1266–72.

59. Burtscher M. Effects of living at higher altitudes on mortality: a narrative review. Aging Dis 2013;5:274–80.

60. Bärtsch P, Swenson ER. Clinical practice: acute high-altitude illnesses. N Engl J Med 2013;368: 2294–302.

61. Brook RD, Rajagopalan S. Particulate matter air pollution and blood pressure. J Am Soc Hypertens 2009;3:332–50.

62. Giorgini P, Di Giosia P, Grassi D, et al. Air pollution exposure and blood pressure: an updated review of the literature. Curr Pharm Des 2015;22:28–51.

63. Brook RD, Rajagopalan S, Pope CA 3rd, et al. Particulate matter air pollution and cardiovascular disease: an Update to the scientific statement from the American Heart Association. Circulation 2010; 121:2331–78.

64. Brook RD, Sun Z, Brook JR, et al. Extreme air pollution conditions adversely affect blood pressure and insulin resistance: the air pollution and cardiometabolic disease study. Hypertension 2016;67:77–85.

65. Rich DQ, Kipen HM, Huang W, et al. Association between changes in air pollution levels during the Beijing Olympics and biomarkers of inflammation and thrombosis in healthy young adults. JAMA 2012;307:2068–78.

66. Liang R, Zhang B, Zhao X, et al. Effect of exposure to PM2.5 on blood pressure: a systematic review and meta-analysis. J Hypertens 2014;32:2130–40.

67. Chen H, Burnett RT, Kwong JC, et al. Spatial association between ambient fine particulate matter and incident hypertension. Circulation 2014;129: 562–9.

68. Coogan PF, White LF, Jerrett M, et al. Air pollution and incidence of hypertension and diabetes mellitus in black women living in Los Angeles. Circulation 2012;125:767–72.

69. Pope CA 3rd, Turner MC, Burnett RT, et al. Relationships between fine particulate air pollution, cardiometabolic disorders, and cardiovascular mortality. Circ Res 2015;116:108–15.

70. Bard RL, Dvonch JT, Kaciroti N, et al. Is acute high-dose secondhand smoke exposure always harmful to microvascular function in healthy adults? Prev Cardiol 2010;13:175–9.

71. Brook RD, Bard RL, Burnett RT, et al. Differences in blood pressure and vascular responses associated with ambient fine particulate matter exposures measured at the personal versus community level. Occup Environ Med 2011;68:224–30.

72. Makrisk TK, Thomapoulous C, Papadopoulous DP, et al. Association of passive smoking with masked hypertension in clinically normotensive nonsmokers. Am J Hypertens 2009;22:853–9.

73. Yarlioglues M, Kaya MG, Ardic I, et al. Acute effects of passive smoking on blood pressure and heart rate in healthy females. Blood Press Monit 2010; 15:251–6.

74. Seki M, Inoue R, Ohkubo T, et al. Association of environmental tobacco smoke exposure with elevated home blood pressure in Japanese women: the Ohasma study. J Hypertens 2010;28:1814–20.

75. Heiss C, Amabile N, lee AC, et al. Brief secondhand smoke exposure depresses endothelial progenitor cell activity and endothelial function. J Am Coll Cardiol 2008;51:1760–71.

76. Alshaarawy O, Xiao J, Shankar A. Association of serum cotinine levels and hypertension in never smokers. Hypertension 2013;61:304–8.

77. Li N, Li Z, Chen S, et al. Effects of passive smoking on hypertension in rural Chinese nonsmoking women. J Hypertens 2015;33:2210–4.

78. Brook RD, Kousha T. Air pollution and emergency Department Visits for Hypertension in Edmonton and Calgary, Canada: a case-crossover study. Am J Hypertens 2015;28:1121–6.

79. Morishita M, Thompson KC, Brook RD. Understanding air pollution and cardiovascular diseases: is it preventable? Curr Cardiovasc Risk Rep 2015;9:30.

80. Jones MR, Barnoya J, Stranges S, et al. Cardiovascular events following smoke-free legislations: an updated systematic review and meta-analysis. Curr Environ Health Rep 2014;1:239–49.

81. Young JH, Chang Y-PC, Kim JD-O, et al. Differential susceptibility to hypertension is due to selection during the out-of-Africa expansion. PLoS Genet 2005;1:e82.

82. Rostand SG. Ultraviolet light may contribute to geographic and racial pressure differences. Hypertension 1997;30:150–6.

83. Rancière F, Lyons JG, Loh VH, et al. Bisphenol A and the risk of cardiometabolic disorders: a systematic review with meta-analysis of the epidemiological evidence. Environ Health 2015;14:46.

84. Trasande L, Attina TM. Association of exposure to di-2-ethylhexylphthalate replacements with increased blood pressure in children and adolescents. Hypertension 2015;66:301–8.

85. Lind L, Lind PM. Can persistent organic pollutants and plastic-associated chemicals cause cardiovascular disease? J Intern Med 2012;271:537–53.

86. Wing S, Horton RA, Rose KM. Air pollution from industrial swine operations and blood pressure of neighboring residents. Environ Health Perspect 2013;121:92–6.

Psychosocial Factors and Hypertension
A Review of the Literature

Adolfo G. Cuevas, PhD[a], David R. Williams, PhD, MPH[b,c,*], Michelle A. Albert, MD, MPH[d]

KEYWORDS

- Hypertension • Psychosocial factors • Health disparities • Race/ethnicity • Review

KEY POINTS

- Hypertension is a leading cause of cardiovascular disease and stroke and this burden falls heavily on black people (African Americans).
- This article reviews recent research on psychosocial factors and hypertension and contextualizes the findings within a health disparities framework.
- This article reveals that psychosocial factors, such as socioeconomic status, stressors (including race-related stressors), and emotional states, may contribute to hypertension risks.
- Future research should investigate how psychosocial factors accumulate over the life course to contribute to hypertension disparities.
- Further research on psychosocial factors and hypertension can enhance the effectiveness of interventions to reduce hypertension risks in ethnic minority patients and communities.

INTRODUCTION

Hypertension is a pervasive problem in the United States, with approximately a third of Americans reporting being diagnosed with hypertension by their physicians or taking antihypertensive medicine.[1] Hypertension is an important risk factor for a variety of health conditions, such as cardiovascular disease, stroke, and kidney failure.[1] Nevertheless, this burden is unevenly distributed in society, with black people having the highest prevalence of hypertension compared with their white counterparts.[1] Despite improvements in increasing the awareness and treatment of hypertension, racial/ethnic differences in hypertension persist.

Growing evidence points to multiple psychological and social factors as contributors to the onset and trajectory of hypertension. Psychosocial factors that induce emotional stress can evoke a physiologic response mediated in part by activation of the sympathetic nervous system, inflammation, and the hypothalamic-pituitary-adrenal axis.[2,3] Repeated activation of this system can result in failing to return to resting blood pressure levels. Psychosocial factors, such as hostility and job strain, have been found to be associated with higher circulating levels of catecholamines, higher cortisol levels, and increased blood pressure over time.[4]

Prior reviews have identified several psychosocial indicators as potential risk factors for the onset

Disclosure Statement: The authors have nothing to disclose.
[a] Department of Social and Behavioral Sciences, Harvard T.H. Chan School of Public Health, Landmark Center, Room 428a, 401 Park Drive, Boston, MA 02215, USA; [b] Department of Social and Behavioral Sciences, Harvard T.H. Chan School of Public Health, 677 Huntington Avenue, 6th Floor, Boston, MA 02115, USA; [c] Department of African and African American Studies, Harvard University, 12 Quincy Street, Cambridge, MA 02138, USA; [d] Division of Cardiology, Department of Medicine, Center for the Study of Adversity and Cardiovascular Disease [NURTURE Center], University of California, San Francisco, 505 Parnassus Avenue, M1177, San Francisco, CA 94143, USA
* Corresponding author.
E-mail address: dwilliam@hsph.harvard.edu

Cardiol Clin 35 (2017) 223–230
http://dx.doi.org/10.1016/j.ccl.2016.12.004
0733-8651/17/© 2017 Elsevier Inc. All rights reserved.

cardiology.theclinics.com

and progression of hypertension.[2,5] This article provides an overview of recent findings related to major psychosocial factors and hypertension. Because of space constraints, emerging work about psychosocial factors (eg, personality, sleep quality[5]) cannot be fully discussed. Nevertheless, in presenting the major factors, this article highlights gaps in the extant literature that contribute to the limited understanding of the social determinants of the persistent racial/ethnic hypertension disparities and discusses directions for future research.

Socioeconomic Status

Socioeconomic status (SES) has long been identified as a risk factor for hypertension. A review by Spruill[2] suggests a complex interaction of social, psychological, and behavioral factors contributing to unequal distribution of diseases. Compared with their high-SES peers, individuals of low SES are more likely to lack sociopolitical power and economic resources, thereby resulting in occupancy of educational, occupational, residential, and recreational environments that are less health enhancing.[6] These factors lead to differential exposures to stressors (eg, unemployment, crime, and violence) and fewer resources (eg, recreation and physical activity) to cope with an accumulation of stressors that combine to contribute to greater risk of hypertension.[2] In a recent meta-analysis, multiple indicators of SES (ie, income, occupation, and education) were associated with an increased risk of hypertension.[7]

SES and race/ethnicity are closely intertwined.[2] Contemporary racial/ethnic categories simultaneously capture unmeasured confounding for biological factors associated with ancestral history and geographic origins; factors linked to current and earlier psychological, social, physical, and chemical environmental exposures; as well as biological adaptation to these exposures.[8] Racial/ethnic differences in SES are large and persistent, and likely contribute to racial/ethnic differences in hypertension. Recent national data reveal that black households earn 59 cents and Hispanics households 70 cents for every dollar of income that white households receive; moreover, black people have only 6 cents and Hispanics 7 cents for every dollar of wealth that white people have.[6]

In addition, because of the persistence of a residual association between race and hypertension after controlling for modifiable risk factors and SES, other unmeasured explanatory factors likely contribute to hypertension disparities.[9] Research suggests that a life-course perspective provides insight into the prolonged impact that early SES

can have on blood pressure. Although most studies taking a life-course perspective are cross-sectional studies, they suggest that the accumulation of stress caused by SES positioning likely promotes health-damaging effects later in life. For instance, low childhood SES and childhood adversity are associated with higher risk of hypertension.[10,11] Slopen and colleagues[12] found that a positive neighborhood context may modify the relationship between childhood adversity and cumulative biological risk in adulthood. Importantly, because evidence suggests that racial/ethnic minorities have higher cumulative stress than white people,[13] further research is needed to examine the extent to which race/ethnicity may moderate the association between the accumulation of stressors over the life course and hypertension.

Race-Related/Ethnicity-Related Stress

Discrimination

Growing attention is paid to the ways in which race-related/ethnicity-related aspects of social experience may adversely affect health, such as discrimination.[9] Discrimination can erode an individual's health through negative psychological and physiologic responses and untoward health maintenance and behaviors.[14] Nevertheless, the literature on discrimination and hypertension is riddled with inconsistent findings, partly caused by measurement issues and the shortage of longitudinal studies.[9,15] For example, research from the Jackson Heart Study found that lifetime discrimination and the burden of discrimination were each modestly associated with increased hypertension prevalence.[16] However, no association was observed between hypertension and a measure of current everyday discrimination. It is plausible that reports of current exposure to minor instances of discrimination might be related to short-term measured blood pressure change, whereas lifetime measures might more aptly capture the cumulative effect of discriminatory exposure on blood pressure risk over time.[16] Not surprisingly, chronic discrimination is more consistently associated with ambulatory blood pressure than with resting clinic blood pressure.[17]

Pathways through which discrimination might affect hypertension risk are multiple. Although prior research indicates that black people are more likely than white people to have a blunted blood pressure decline during sleep, emerging studies reveal that exposure to discrimination contributes to the increased levels of blood pressure and lack of blood pressure decrease among black people at night.[14] Sleep disturbances are also related to hypertension risk. Moreover, a recent review indicates that discrimination is positively associated with reported sleep difficulties, insomnia, and fatigue, thereby influencing hypertension risk.[18] In other research, threat of exposure to discrimination versus actual exposure also affects hypertension risk, possibly via heightened vigilance.[19] Experiences of discrimination have also been associated with lower levels of adherence and follow-up for multiple health conditions, and, if this pattern is also true of hypertension, it could contribute to greater severity and poorer course of hypertension.[14] In light of these points, future studies should consider the multiple dimensions of discrimination and conditions that adversely affect blood pressure.[17]

Goal-striving stress
There are other, more novel race-related risk factors that may also play a role. Goal-striving stress is a measure of thwarted aspirations. It is typically operationalized as the discrepancy between aspirations and achievement, weighted by the subjective probability of success and the level of disappointment experienced if goals are not reached.[20] Analyses of a large national sample revealed that higher levels of goal-striving stress were associated with the prevalence of self-reported hypertension among white Americans, African Americans, and Caribbean black people, and race/ethnicity did not moderate the relationship between goal-striving stress and hypertension.[20] Longitudinal research is needed to enhance the understanding of the timing of the development of goal-striving stress and how exposure and response to it may influence the onset and course of hypertension disparities. Relatedly, John Henryism, an active predisposition to succeed against all odds, is associated with high blood pressure among persons who lack the resources to facilitate success.[21] Research is needed to better understand the conditions under which psychological risk factors and coping mechanisms such as goal-striving stress and John Henryism can affect the development and course of hypertension and the behavioral and biological mechanisms through which these processes occur.[21]

Internalized racism
Self-stereotyping (or internalized racism) has been identified as another mechanism by which racism might adversely affect health. Limited research indicates a positive association between internalized racism and multiple health outcomes, including overweight/obesity and blood pressure.[14] Other data show that internalized racism

interacts with discrimination to predict increased risk of hypertension,[22] such that, in a sample of 91 African American men, increased hypertension risk was only evident for African American men who scored high both on discrimination and anti-black bias.

Stereotype threat is a term describing the activation of negative stereotypes in members of a stigmatized group that creates reactions, anxieties, and expectations that adversely affect psychological functioning and health.[23] For example, in the work by Blascovich and colleagues,[24] physiologic arousal triggered by stereotype threat is associated with greater increases in blood pressure among African Americans than in European American students. Stereotype threat is also purported to trigger increases in anxiety and impairment of decision-making and self-regulation processes in a manner that increases aggressive behavior and overeating.[25] Stereotype threat may be indirectly related to hypertension through weight changes and modulation of the neural hormonal system.[26,27] In addition, stereotype threat can lead affected persons to delay seeking needed medical care, and to have poor adherence to recommended therapies and generally poor patient-provider relationships.[14]

Other Sources of Stress

Occupational stress
Previous research suggests that working conditions that induce stress are associated with increased risk of hypertension.[2,28] Occupational stressors can include hostile work environments (eg, threatened, bullied, or harassed by anyone while on the job), work insecurity (eg, worried about becoming unemployed), time pressures, work hazards, and other work conditions (eg, sedentary tasks, uncontrollable tasks).[28] High job strain/stress (high job demand and low job control) is independently associated with hypertension, ambulatory blood pressure increase, and cardiovascular disease risk.[29–31]

Occupations with high job demand and low job control (eg, servers and clerks) are commonly overrepresented among ethnic minorities.[32] However, the relationship between job strain and hypertension has been mixed, particularly for black people. For instance, low decisional control has been found to be related to increased blood pressure reactivity among black people.[33,34] However, a recent study using Health and Retirement Study data found no association between high job strain (as well as workplace discrimination) and hypertension among African Americans.[35] Considering the paucity of epidemiologic studies examining the relationship between work-related stressors and hypertension among racial/ethnic minority workers, these results require replication using national data sets. Furthermore, other job strain domains, especially those that may be more salient for ethnic minorities (eg, stressors linked to unemployment and underemployment, job conflict, or financial strain caused by low wages) should be explored in this area of research.[35]

An important direction for future research is to more comprehensively assess the broad range of stressors that might affect hypertension risk. For example, with regard to work stress, studies need to go beyond assessing high demand and low control and assess conditions in work environments that are likely to vary by race, such as physical and chemical environmental hazards and occupational stressors linked to injury risk.[8] Because research studies have assessed only a few domains of stressors, systematic attention needs to be given to understanding the contribution of a broader range of living conditions that could increase hypertension risk, including incarceration, which disproportionately affects black people. For example, the Coronary Artery Risk Development in Young Adults (CARDIA) study found that incarceration was associated with increased risk of incident hypertension 3 years later and greater end-organ damage related to hypertension.[36] Incarceration is a type of stressful experience that exacerbates social disadvantage by placing many people on a pathway of low education, poor job prospects, and low income. These examples highlight the need to fully characterize all aspects of the social context that can negatively affect hypertension risk.

Emotional States

High levels of anxiety and depression symptoms are common in adults, often comorbid with chronic illnesses such as hypertension, and can have deleterious effects on individual health and quality of life. A meta-analysis of prospective studies found that depressive symptoms predict a 42% increased risk of hypertension.[37] Similar to the findings for depressive symptoms, a meta-analysis of prospective studies found that anxiety symptoms were an independent risk factor for incident hypertension.[38] However, many studies are limited by the lack of control for confounding factors, such as risk behaviors and related psychological factors (eg, anger), which may attenuate observed relationships between these emotional states and hypertension. Future research should adjust for all related factors to

accurately assess the independent contribution of depression and anxiety to hypertension.

Consistent with prior research, recent evidence continues to document that anger and hostility are associated with increased hypertension risk.[39] For example, using data from the Heart Strategies Concentrating On Risk Evaluation, researchers noted that high levels of hostility are associated with an attenuated nocturnal decline in blood pressure among black people and white people.[40] Most research in this area has been limited to white men,[39] which also limits the understanding of racial and gender differences in levels of exposures to these risk factors and the extent to which the effects of such exposures vary by social group. In addition, as noted by Trudel-Fitzgerald and colleagues,[39] few prospective studies with up-to-date methodology have been conducted within the last decade. However, longitudinal analyses from the Jackson Heart Study show that African Americans with high anger-out (expressed rather than repressed anger) scores have a 20% increased risk of blood pressure progression compared with African Americans with low anger-out scores.[41] Prospective studies are needed to identify the independent effect of anger (both experience and expression) on blood pressure in diverse population samples.

Trudel-Fitzgerald and colleagues[39] introduced 2 emerging psychosocial factors that should be considered within the larger literature of emotional states and hypertension: positive psychological well-being (PPWB) and emotion regulation. Growing evidence suggests that PPWB, such as optimism, life satisfaction, and emotional vitality, is positively associated with hypertension and cardiovascular health risk factors (eg, physical activity).[39,42] However, the link between PPWB and hypertension has not been well established because of methodological and measurement issues (eg, the heterogeneity of hypertension measurements).[39] Similarly, although vitality predicts hypertension onset,[43] further research using a broader range of PPWB domains is needed to fully understand the influence of PPWB on hypertension. In addition, emotion regulation, which refers to the monitoring of a person's emotional experiences and responses, may also influence physical health, including hypertension risk, but research in this area is limited by lack of diversity and longitudinal studies.[39]

Social Relationships

Social relationships serve as sources of emotional support (eg, empathy), informational support, and instrumental support. These positive aspects of social ties have been shown to directly enhance health and to reduce the negative effects of stressful experiences on health by enhancing the capacity of individuals to cope with stress. These processes are also likely to affect hypertension risk.[2,5] For example, a study using National Health Interview Survey data found that both emotional support and social integration were independently associated with decreased odds of hypertension.[44] The study also suggested that emotional support and social integration seemed to buffer the adverse effects of low SES on hypertension.[44] However, the interrelationships between race/ethnicity, hypertension, and social relationships have not been clearly elucidated. The limited available research in this area indicates that race/ethnic differences in hypertension are reduced among people who receive social support, compared with those who do not receive any form of support.[45] Although this study did not find an interaction effect between marital status and ethnicity in predicting hypertension, the potential contribution of marital status, a key component of social relationships, deserves more concerted attention in research on hypertension. Marital status, similar to other measures of social ties, can have both positive and negative effects on health, particularly hypertension.[2] However, inadequate attention has been given to examining the association between marital relationships and other types of social ties and blood pressure among ethnic minorities and their potential contribution to hypertension disparities. This omission is especially important given that black people are less likely to be married than white people and it is currently unclear whether other social relationships compensate for the lower levels of marital ties among black people.

Other Research Priorities

The role of genetics in racial/ethnic differences in hypertension remains as an ongoing debate. Although evidence suggests that polymorphisms in the APOL 1 (Apolipoprotein L1) gene may contribute to hypertension propensity in black people,[46] socioenvironmental influences are critical. For example, research shows that, although black people in the United States have higher rates of hypertension than white people in European countries such as Sweden and Italy, they have lower prevalence levels than white people in other countries such as Germany and Finland.[47] Increasing evidence also suggests that epigenetic modifications, caused by, for instance, childhood development or chemical exposure, are important contributors to the development of hypertension.[48] However, there are only a limited number of studies of epigenetic changes linked to hypertension risk factors, and only blood rather than the effector tissues have been examined, limiting the present understanding of the contribution of DNA methylation to high blood pressure.[48] Future studies should consider examining both blood methylation and effector tissues to more fully understand the contribution of epigenetics to hypertension disparities.

Another issue of concern relates to the lack of attention to, or the assumption of, nonheterogeneity within ethnic groups. Studies of black people tend to cluster immigrant African and Caribbean black people with US-born black people, regardless of acculturation status and country of origin. White people are also viewed as monolithic with, little attention given to recent eastern European immigrants or groups from North Africa and the Middle East that are grouped into the official 'White' category in the United States. Similarly, studies cluster Hispanic people, regardless of acculturation status, race, and country of origin, potentially diluting the measurement of the differential impact of environment on hypertension risk. Greater acculturation is associated with increased hypertension risk, independent of age, gender, race/ethnicity, education, smoking, alcohol, physical activity, body mass index, and diabetes.[49] In addition, there is disconcertingly little research about the determinants of hypertension risk in America's indigenous populations (Native Hawaiians and other Pacific Islanders and American Indians and Alaskan Natives), despite a higher prevalence of hypertension in these groups compared with other ethnic groups.[50] An enhanced understanding of psychosocial risks and resources associated with the historical and contemporary conditions in which these groups live, learn, work, play, and worship can facilitate the identification of culturally sensitive intervention strategies for hypertension.[51]

In addition, although other psychosocial factors, such as sleep disturbances, were not covered in depth in this article, their exclusion does not diminish the value of their inclusion in future research. For example, sleep quality and certain personality factors (eg, neuroticism) may contribute to hypertension risk.[5] However, similar to several other factors discussed, much of the evidence comes from studies of white people, which restricts understanding as to how they may contribute to existing hypertension disparities.

Psychosocial Interventions

At present, lifestyle modifications remain the most effective interventions to reduce hypertension risk.

Lifestyle modification, including increasing physical activity, reducing alcohol intake, and reducing sodium intake, through programs such as Dietary Approaches to Stop Hypertension (DASH), reduces hypertension risk.[52] Although lifestyle modification is important, especially for black and Hispanic people, who have high rates of overweight/obesity and physical inactivity, making lifestyle changes is challenging for disadvantaged populations in the absence of comprehensive efforts to address the underlying social conditions that give rise to the risk behaviors in the first place.[53] Socially disadvantaged groups face a multitude of stressors, coupled with limited resources, which can limit the effectiveness of interventions that are narrowly focused on the behavior without attention to the social conditions that initiate and sustain them.[54]

Stress and depression management/interventions should be complementary additions to lifestyle modification. Evidence suggests that stress-reducing interventions, such as transcendental meditation, decreases diastolic and systolic blood pressures.[55,56] To address race-related stressors, such as racial discrimination, Lewis and colleagues[57] highlighted promising interventions that can reduce the effects of discrimination on health, such as religious involvement, values affirmation, forgiveness, and racism countermarketing.

Interventions addressing SES disparities at the neighborhood level are also important.[8] Racial/ethnic and SES segregation in particular can increase the risk of morbidity and mortality through limited socioeconomic mobility, restrained access to health resources, exposure to toxins and environmental stressors (eg, violence), and weakened neighborhood social capital.[8] Further research priority needs to be given to understanding the complex influence of poverty and racial segregation on health. Policies and interventions that improve neighborhood and housing quality, increase household income, and improve education can help to improve the health of socially disadvantaged populations.[54] For example, randomized housing interventions (eg, Moving to Opportunity) showed that moving poor residents from high-poverty public housing apartments to lower-poverty neighborhood environments, with no health interventions, reduced obesity and diabetes risk 10 to 15 years later,[56] an action that likely also influences blood pressure outcomes.

SUMMARY

Understanding hypertension disparities remains an important and complex issue in human health. There is a great need for further research to better understand and effectively address the role of psychosocial factors in the disproportionate burden of hypertension on racial/ethnic minorities. Taking a life-course perspective that captures the accumulation of risks over time may help address some of the questions about the effect of psychosocial factors on hypertension risk that still puzzle researchers. In addition, future research should address methodological limitations of the existing literature, including identifying and controlling for a broad set of core confounding factors, using appropriately accurate measures of blood pressure (eg, self-reported hypertension vs ambulatory blood pressure), and doing more longitudinal research. Addressing such issues could help disentangle existing complexities and generate new insights that can potentially greatly improve the effectiveness of interventions that seek to reduce hypertension disparities.

REFERENCES

1. Mozaffarian D, Benjamin EJ, Go AS, et al. Executive summary: heart disease and stroke Statistics—2016 update. Circulation 2016;133(4):447–54.
2. Spruill TM. Chronic psychosocial stress and hypertension. Curr Hypertens Rep 2010;12(1):10–6.
3. Black PH, Garbutt LD. Stress, inflammation and cardiovascular disease. J Psychosom Res 2002;52(1):1–23.
4. Everson-Rose SA, Lewis TT. Psychosocial factors and cardiovascular diseases. Annu Rev Public Health 2005;26(1):469–500.
5. Cuffee Y, Ogedegbe C, Williams NJ, et al. Psychosocial risk factors for hypertension: an update of the literature. Curr Hypertens Rep 2014;16(10):483.
6. Williams DR, Priest N, Anderson N. Understanding associations between race, socioeconomic status and health: patterns and prospects. Health Psychol 2016;35(4):407–11.
7. Leng B, Jin Y, Li G, et al. Socioeconomic status and hypertension: a meta-analysis. J Hypertens 2015;33(2):221–9.
8. Williams DR, Mohammed SA, Leavell J, et al. Race, socioeconomic status, and health: complexities, ongoing challenges, and research opportunities. Ann N Y Acad Sci 2010;1186:69–101.
9. Dolezsar CM, McGrath JJ, Herzig AJM, et al. Perceived racial discrimination and hypertension: a comprehensive systematic review. Health Psychol 2014;33(1):20–34.
10. James SA, Van Hoewyk J, Belli RF, et al. Life-course socioeconomic position and hypertension in African American men: the Pitt County study. Am J Public Health 2006;96(5):812–7.
11. Crowell JA, Davis CR, Joung KE, et al. Metabolic pathways link childhood adversity to elevated blood

pressure in midlife adults. Obes Res Clin Pract 2016;10(5):580–8.

12. Slopen N, Non A, Williams DR, et al. Childhood adversity, adult neighborhood context, and cumulative biological risk for chronic diseases in adulthood. Psychosom Med 2014;76(7):481–9.

13. Sternthal M, Slopen N, Williams DR. Racial disparities in health: how much does stress really matter? Du Bois Review 2011;8(1):95–113.

14. Williams DR, Mohammed SA. Racism and health I: pathways and scientific evidence. Am Behav Sci 2013;57(8). http://dx.doi.org/10.1177/0002764213 487340.

15. Cuffee YL, Hargraves JL, Allison J. Exploring the association between reported discrimination and hypertension among African Americans: a systematic review. Ethn Dis 2012;22(4):422–31.

16. Sims M, Diez-Roux AV, Dudley A, et al. Perceived discrimination and hypertension among African Americans in the Jackson Heart Study. Am J Public Health 2012;102(Suppl 2):S258–65.

17. Brondolo E, Love EE, Pencille M, et al. Racism and hypertension: a review of the empirical evidence and implications for clinical practice. Am J Hypertens 2011;24(5):518–29.

18. Slopen N, Lewis TT, Williams DR. Discrimination and sleep: a systematic review. Sleep Med 2016; 18:88–95.

19. Hicken MT, Lee H, Morenoff J, et al. Racial/ethnic disparities in hypertension prevalence: reconsidering the role of chronic stress. Am J Public Health 2014;104(1):117–23.

20. Sellers SL, Neighbors HW, Zhang R, et al. The impact of goal-striving stress on physical health of white Americans, African Americans, and Caribbean blacks. Ethn Dis 2012;22(1):21–8.

21. Bennett GG, Merritt MM, Sollers JJ III, et al. Stress, coping, and health outcomes among African-Americans: a review of the John Henryism hypothesis. Psychol Health 2004;19(3):369–83.

22. Chae DH, Nuru-Jeter AM, Adler NE. Implicit racial bias as a moderator of the association between racial discrimination and hypertension: a study of midlife African American men. Psychosom Med 2012;74(9):961–4.

23. Steele CM. A threat in the air. How stereotypes shape intellectual identity and performance. Am Psychol 1997;52(6):613–29.

24. Blascovich J, Spencer SJ, Quinn D, et al. African Americans and high blood pressure: the role of stereotype threat. Psychol Sci 2001;12(3):225–9.

25. Inzlicht M, Kang SK. Stereotype threat spillover: how coping with threats to social identity affects aggression, eating, decision making, and attention. J Pers Soc Psychol 2010;99(3):467–81.

26. Meyer N, Richter SH, Schreiber RS, et al. The unexpected effects of beneficial and adverse social experiences during adolescence on anxiety and aggression and their modulation by genotype. Front Behav Neurosci 2016;10:97.

27. Rana S, Pugh PC, Katz E, et al. Independent effects of early-life experience and trait aggression on cardiovascular function. Am J Physiol Regul Integr Comp Physiol 2016;311(2):R272–86.

28. Rosenthal T, Alter A. Occupational stress and hypertension. J Am Soc Hypertens 2012;6(1):2–22.

29. Babu GR, Jotheeswaran AT, Mahapatra T, et al. Is hypertension associated with job strain? A meta-analysis of observational studies. Occup Environ Med 2014;71(3):220–7.

30. Landsbergis PA, Dobson M, Koutsouras G, et al. Job strain and ambulatory blood pressure: a meta-analysis and systematic review. Am J Public Health 2013;103(3):e61–71.

31. Slopen N, Glynn RJ, Buring JE, et al. Job strain, job insecurity, and incident cardiovascular disease in the Women's Health Study: results from a 10-year prospective study. PLoS One 2012;7(7):e40512.

32. Buchanan S, Vossenas P, Krause N, et al. Occupational injury disparities in the US hotel industry. Am J Ind Med 2010;53(2):116–25.

33. Thomas KS, Nelesen RA, Ziegler MG, et al. Job strain, ethnicity, and sympathetic nervous system activity. Hypertension 2004;44(6):891–6.

34. Curtis AB, James SA, Raghunathan TE, et al. Job strain and blood pressure in African Americans: the Pitt County study. Am J Public Health 1997; 87(8):1297–302.

35. Mezuk B, Kershaw KN, Hudson D, et al. Job strain, workplace discrimination, and hypertension among older workers: the health and retirement study. Race Soc Probl 2011;3(1):38–50.

36. Wang E, Pletcher M, Lin F, et al. Incarceration, incident hypertension, and access to health care: findings from the Coronary Artery Risk Development in Young Adults (CARDIA) study. Arch Intern Med 2009;169(7):687–93.

37. Meng L, Chen D, Yang Y, et al. Depression increases the risk of hypertension incidence: a meta-analysis of prospective cohort studies. J Hypertens 2012; 30(5):842–51.

38. Pan Y, Cai W, Cheng Q, et al. Association between anxiety and hypertension: a systematic review and meta-analysis of epidemiological studies. Neuropsychiatr Dis Treat 2015;11:1121–30.

39. Trudel-Fitzgerald C, Gilsanz P, Mittleman MA, et al. Dysregulated blood pressure: can regulating emotions help? Curr Hypertens Rep 2015;17(12):1–9.

40. Mezick EJ, Matthews KA, Hall M, et al. Low life purpose and high hostility are related to an attenuated decline in nocturnal blood pressure. Health Psychol 2010;29(2):196–204.

41. Ford CD, Sims M, Higginbotham JC, et al. Psychosocial factors are associated with blood pressure

progression among African Americans in the Jackson Heart Study. Am J Hypertens 2016;29(8): 913–24.

42. Boehm JK, Kubzansky LD. The heart's content: the association between positive psychological well-being and cardiovascular health. Psychol Bull 2012;138(4):655–91.

43. Trudel-Fitzgerald C, Boehm JK, Kivimaki M, et al. Taking the tension out of hypertension: a prospective study of psychological well being and hypertension. J Hypertens 2014;32(6):1222–8.

44. Gorman BK, Sivaganesan A. The role of social support and integration for understanding socioeconomic disparities in self-rated health and hypertension. Soc Sci Med 2007;65(5):958–75.

45. Bell CN, Thorpe RJ, LaVeist TA. Race/ethnicity and hypertension: the role of social support. Am J Hypertens 2010;23(5):534–40.

46. Freedman BI, Murea M. Target organ damage in African American hypertension: role of APOL1. Curr Hypertens Rep 2012;14(1):21–8.

47. Cooper RS, Wolf-Maier K, Luke A, et al. An international comparative study of blood pressure in populations of European vs. African descent. BMC Med 2005;3:2.

48. Wise IA, Charchar FJ. Epigenetic modifications in essential hypertension. Int J Mol Sci 2016;17(4):451.

49. Teppala S, Shankar A, Ducatman A. The association between acculturation and hypertension in a multi-ethnic sample of US adults. J Am Soc Hypertens 2010;4(5):236–43.

50. Centers for Disease Control and Prevention (CDC). Health status of American Indians compared with other racial/ethnic minority populations–selected states, 2001-2002. MMWR Morb Mortal Wkly Rep 2003;52(47):1148–52.

51. Kaholokula JK, Iwane MK, Nacapoy AH. Effects of perceived racism and acculturation on hypertension in native Hawaiians. Hawaii Med J 2010; 69(5 suppl 2):11–5.

52. Schwingshackl L, Hoffmann G. Diet quality as assessed by the Healthy Eating Index, the Alternate Healthy Eating Index, the Dietary Approaches to Stop Hypertension score, and health outcomes: a systematic review and meta-analysis of cohort studies. J Acad Nutr Diet 2015;115(5):780–800.e5.

53. Brook RD, Appel LJ, Rubenfire M, et al. Beyond medications and diet: alternative approaches to lowering blood pressure a scientific statement from the American Heart Association. Hypertension 2013;61(6):1360–83.

54. Williams DR, Mohammed SA. Racism and health II: a needed research agenda for effective interventions. Am Behav Sci 2013;57(8). http://dx.doi.org/10.1177/0002764213487341.

55. Rainforth MV, Schneider RH, Nidich SI, et al. Stress reduction programs in patients with elevated blood pressure: a systematic review and meta-analysis. Curr Hypertens Rep 2008;9(6):520–8.

56. Ludwig J, Sanbonmatsu L, Gennetian L, et al. Neighborhoods, obesity, and diabetes — a randomized social experiment. N Engl J Med 2011;365(16): 1509–19.

57. Lewis TT, Cogburn CD, Williams DR. Self-reported experiences of discrimination and health: scientific advances, ongoing controversies, and emerging issues. Annu Rev Clin Psychol 2015;11(1):407–40.

Management of Essential Hypertension

Keith C. Ferdinand, MD[a],*, Samar A. Nasser, PhD, MPH, PA-C[b]

KEYWORDS

- Essential hypertension • Pharmacotherapy • Lifestyle modification • African American
- Elderly • Goals

KEY POINTS

- Prevalence of essential hypertension is widespread in the United States and highest in African Americans. Racial/ethnic US minorities have lower hypertension control rates compared with non-Hispanic whites.
- Therapeutic lifestyle modifications are essential for all patients with essential hypertension, as a first step and also in conjunction with pharmacotherapy. The initial recommended drug therapy for patients without compelling conditions includes thiazide-type diuretics, calcium channel blockers (CCBs), angiotensin-converting enzyme inhibitors (ACEis) or angiotensin receptor blockers (ARBs).
- African Americans may have a better response to thiazide-type diuretic and CCBs as first-step therapy for blood pressure (BP) reduction and cardiovascular (CV) outcomes compared with ACEis or ARBs, only if there are no compelling indications for these other antihypertensive agents.
- Beta-blockers in older patients are less effective first-step agents for BP control and CV risk reduction, unless compelling indications, such as post–myocardial infarction status, are present.
- In multiple recent guidelines, the BP goal for most patients with essential hypertension is less than 140/90 mm Hg. More intensive goals may be recommended in future guidelines for high-risk patients, including persons with diabetes mellitus and in elderly patients, based on recent randomized clinical trial evidence.

INTRODUCTION

The present evidence-based treatment of essential hypertension is a critical intervention in decreasing cardiovascular (CV) morbidity and mortality.[1] The World Health Organization considers elevated blood pressure (BP) as the most important risk factor for death and disability worldwide, affecting more than 1 billion individuals and causing an estimated 9.4 million deaths every year.[2]

A contemporary meta-analysis of 123 studies with 613,815 hypertensive participants noted for every 10-mm Hg reduction in systolic BP (SBP), there is a significant reduction of the risk of major CV disease (CVD) events (relative risk 0.80, 95% confidence interval [CI] 0.77–0.83), coronary heart disease (CHD) (0.83, 0.78–0.88), stroke (0.73, 0.68–0.77), and heart failure (HF) (0.72, 0.67–0.78). Importantly, although the effect on renal failure was not significant (0.95, 0.84–1.07), there was a significant (13%) reduction in all-cause mortality (0.87, 0.84–0.91).[3]

In consideration of the preponderance of present data, BP lowering significantly reduces CV risk across various baseline BP levels and comorbidities, especially in high-risk patients. There is

Disclosure: Grant/research: Boehringer Ingelheim; consultant: Amgen, Sanofi, Boehringer Ingelheim, Eli Lilly (K.C. Ferdinand). No conflicts of interest (S.A. Nasser).

[a] Tulane Heart and Vascular Institute, Tulane University School of Medicine, 1430 Tulane Avenue, #8548, New Orleans, LA 70112, USA; [b] Department of Clinical Research & Leadership, School of Medicine and Health Sciences, The George Washington University, 2100 Pennsylvania Avenue, Northwest, Suite 354, Washington, DC 20006, USA
* Corresponding author.
E-mail address: kferdina@tulane.edu

consensus in modern guidelines for treating adults with essential hypertension to a goal of less than 140/90 mm Hg. However, based on emerging evidence, there may be increasingly strong support for lowering SBP goals to perhaps less than 130 mm Hg or lower, especially in high-risk patients, including those with a history of CVD, CHD, chronic kidney disease (CKD), stroke, diabetes mellitus (DM), and the elderly. (SPRINT 39)

ESSENTIAL HYPERTENSION IDENTIFICATION, PREVALENCE, AND CONTROL

The generally accepted classification of BP is based on the average of 2 or more properly measured, seated BP readings on each of 2 or more office visits (**Table 1**).

Patients with prehypertension are at increased risk for progression to hypertension, and those in the 130 to 139/80 to 89 mm Hg BP range are at twice the risk to develop hypertension as compared with those with lower values.[4] Presently, stages 2 and 3 hypertension have been combined into stage 2.

The auscultatory or practitioner-determined oscillometric method with a manual cuff is the most common technique in clinical practice and was used in most clinical trials of antihypertensive therapy. In contrast, automated oscillometric BP (AOBP) was used in the Systolic Blood Pressure Intervention Trial (SPRINT) which is a recent landmark trial that may impact recommendations on BP assessment and goals in future evidence-based guidelines. (SPRINT 39) The AOBP technique takes multiple consecutive readings with patients resting alone in a room and is infrequently used in clinical practice A current edition of UpToDate states: "In general, systolic pressure readings are 5 to 10 mm Hg lower with AOBP than with manual (auscultatory) measurement."[5] That should be in quotation marks if it stays.

A recent review compares office BP with manual AOBP and confirms unattended automated BP may elicit lower BP readings than attended BP measurements.[6]

The treatment of essential hypertension is the most common reason for adult clinical visits and for the use of prescription drugs in the United States.[7] The most recent US data available from the National Health and Nutrition Examination Survey from 2011 to 2014 confirm that hypertension remains a public health challenge because of its direct impact on the risk of CVD and renal disease. Moreover, the prevalence of hypertension in adults varies across race/ethnicity. Non-Hispanic blacks have the highest rates of hypertension prevalence nationally (40.8% for men, 41.5% for women). The rates are significantly lower for non-Hispanic whites, non-Hispanic Asians, and Hispanics, in both men and women (**Fig. 1**).[8]

Furthermore, the prevalence of controlled hypertension varies across race/ethnicity with non-Hispanic whites having a 55.7% control rate (53.8% in men, 59.1% in women), which is higher than that seen in racial/ethnic minorities.

- African Americans (AAs): 48.5% overall control rate
- Non-Hispanic Asians: 43.5% overall control rate
- Hispanics: 47.4% overall control rate[8]

HYPERTENSION IN AFRICAN AMERICANS

Hypertension in AAs is the most powerful cause for disparities in CV and renal morbidity and mortality in this population as compared with non-Hispanic whites. Black men and women are more likely to die of heart disease and stroke, which are not only the leading causes of death for all Americans but account for the largest proportion of inequality in life expectancy between whites and blacks. These unacceptable disparities persist despite the existence of low-cost, highly effective preventative treatment specifically for the lowering of BP.[10]

There are several unique aspects of hypertension in US blacks compared with whites, which include

- Earlier onset
- Higher average BPs
- Increased incidence of target organ damage, including left ventricular hypertrophy (LVH), HF, impaired renal function, CKD with end-stage renal disease (ESRD), CHD mortality, peripheral arterial disease, and retinopathy

Table 1
Classification of blood pressure based on the Joint National Committee 7

Category	SBP (mm Hg)		DBP (mm Hg)
Normal	<120	And	<80
Prehypertension	120–139	Or	80–89
Hypertension, stage 1	140–159	Or	90–99
Hypertension, stage 2	≥160	Or	≥100

From National High Blood Pressure Education Program. The seventh report of the joint national committee on prevention, detection, evaluation, and treatment of high blood pressure, 2004. Available at: http://www.ncbi.nlm. nih.gov/books/NBK9630/. Accessed June 5, 2016; with permission.

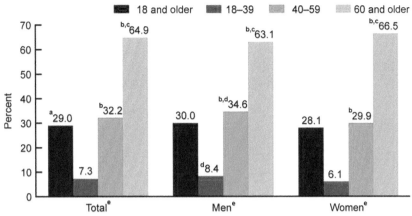

Fig. 1. The prevalence of hypertension in the United States among adults aged 18 years and older, by sex and age (2011–2014). [a] Crude estimates are 31.3% for total, 31.0% for men, and 31.5% for women. [b] Significant difference from age group 18 to 39 years. [c] Significant difference from age group 40 to 59 years. [d] Significant difference from women for same age group. [e] Significant linear trend. Note: Estimates for the 18 years and older category were age adjusted by the direct method to the 2000 US census population using age group 18 to 39 years, 40 to 59 years, and 60 years and older; see reference.[9] (From Yoon SS, Fryar CD, Carroll MD. Hypertension prevalence and control among adults: United States, 2011-2014. NCHS Data Brief No. 220. In: National Center for Health Statistics. 2015. Available at: http://www.cdc.gov/nchs/products/databriefs/db220.htm. Accessed June 5, 2016; with permission; and CDC/NCHS, National Health and Nutrition Examination Survey, 2011-2014.)

In fact, hypertension prevalence among AAs is among the highest in the world, with US blacks having a higher average BP compared with whites.[9,11]

Overall in AAs, various forms of CVD that manifest higher incidence include myocardial infarction (MI) and heart disease, especially in the younger ages; peripheral arterial disease; and HF, which in the black population is more often due to hypertension than coronary artery disease (CAD). The rates of ESRD are also disproportionate in AAs, in part related to the effects of widespread and poorly controlled hypertension in addition to DM.[12] Although apolipoprotein L1 high-risk genotype is present in approximately 13% of blacks in the United States, and acts as a risk factor for kidney function decline in populations with CKD, the high variability in estimated glomerular filtration rate (eGFR) decline among blacks with and without the APOL1 suggests a primary screening tool high-risk genotype population-based screening is not yet justified.

The avoidable death from heart disease and stroke in national data are much higher for blacks than race/sex-matched whites. Black females have a rate of avoidable death from heart disease, stroke, hypertension, and CVD similar to that seen with white males. Specifically, as it relates to the age-adjusted hypertension death rates, AAs, for more than a decade, have had death rates (per 100,000) twice that seen in the general population (**Fig. 2**).[13]

In consequence of disparate hypertension, US life expectancy is unfortunately persistently disproportionate, with black males having the shortest life expectancy and black females having a life expectancy more similar to that of white males than white females.[14]

In consideration of these higher rates of heart disease and stroke morbidity and mortality, the 2013 guidelines from the American College of Cardiology (ACC)/American Heart Association (AHA) for the treatment of blood cholesterol to reduce atherosclerotic risk give higher consideration of risk estimation in AAs.[15]

UNIQUE CONSIDERATIONS OF TREATMENT OF HYPERTENSION IN AFRICAN AMERICANS

In AAs, potential physiologic and hemodynamic determinants may affect the benefits of first-step or initial therapy with thiazide-type diuretics and calcium channel blockers (CCBs) as compared with beta-blockers, angiotensin-converting enzyme inhibitors (ACEis), and angiotensin receptor blockers (ARBs). The potential determinants of hypertension in AAs compared with non-Hispanic whites include the following:

The author considers these general statements later as studied, well-known, and accepted concepts. The author would like to modify the overweight/obesity greater than 50% and keep the others with cite from his review without detailed cites for each statement. The extra labor but no elucidation of new concepts by seeking individual citations.

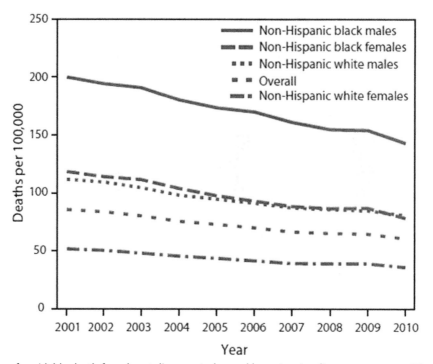

Fig. 2. Rates of avoidable death from heart disease, stroke, and hypertensive disease among non-Hispanic blacks and whites by sex in the United States from 2001 to 2010. (*From* Centers for Disease Control and Prevention (CDC). Vital signs: avoidable deaths from heart disease, stroke, and hypertensive disease — United States, 2001–2010. MMWR Morb Mortal Wkly Rep 2013;6;62(35):724.)

- Overweight and obesity with a body mass index (BMI) of 30 or greater, which affects greater than 50% of AA women
- Higher salt sensitivity
- Low levels of plasma renin
- Abnormal vascular function (sympathetic over activity)
- Attenuated nocturnal decrease in BP
- Greater comorbidity (especially DM)
- Inactivity
- Positive family history

Specifically in the black population, thiazide-type diuretics and CCBs are recommended drugs for initial therapy versus ACEis, ARBs, or beta-blockers, if there are no compelling indications.

The use of ACEis or ARBs in blacks is more effective when combined with thiazide-type diuretics and CCBs. This approach removes any racial differences in BP lowering. The initiation of an ACEi, although decreasing angiotensin II production, may also increase bradykinin levels. This increase may result in regional vasodilatation and an increase in vascular permeability leading to angioedema and may occur even long after the initiation of therapy. In the Antihypertensive and Lipid Lowering Treatment to Prevent Heart Attack Trial (ALLHAT), angioedema was 3 times more common in blacks; this has been reported in other data.[16]

THERAPEUTIC LIFESTYLE MODIFICATIONS: A REQUIRED FIRST STEP IN THE TREATMENT OF ESSENTIAL HYPERTENSION

Essential hypertension is accurately also categorized as primary hypertension, in view of the lack of a clear identifiable cause or single pathogenesis. Greater than 90% of patients commonly treated for hypertension are essential or primary in origin, likely because of the results of multiple, poorly characterized genetic and environmental factors.

The modifiable lifestyle risk factors for essential hypertension most clearly confirmed include the following:

- Obesity
- High sodium intake
- Insufficient physical activity
- Excessive alcohol consumption

Nonmodifiable factors also play important contributing roles, specifically the following:

- Age
- Race

- Family history, perhaps contributed by yet-undefined genetic factors

These modifiable risk factors for essential primary hypertension are strongly and independently associated with its development, despite the lack of a clear cause for most cases of elevated BP. For instance, the high prevalence and persistent rates of overweight and obesity in the United States clearly have an effect on BP prevalence with non-Hispanic black females having overweight and obesity rates greater than 80%. Obesity may additionally increase rates of heart disease and stroke events and is strongly associated with higher rates of comorbid physician-diagnosed DM, which is more prevalent in non-Hispanic blacks and Hispanics than in whites.[17]

Nevertheless, in addition to adverse lifestyle factors, the social determinants of health have a profound effect on the prevalence and adverse outcomes for CVD, including hypertension. The social determinants include the following:

- Socioeconomic position
- Race/ethnicity
- Social support
- Culture
- Language
- Access to care
- Residential environment[18]

The application of therapeutic lifestyle changes remains the bedrock of hypertension care, especially in patients with milder forms of hypertension, and to assist with BP control along with medication.

EVIDENCE-BASED THERAPEUTIC LIFESTYLE CHANGES

The 2013 ACC/AHA guideline on lifestyle management to reduce CV risk highlights the BP lowering benefits of the Dietary Approaches to Stop Hypertension (DASH) eating plan in both men and women (**Table 2**). Also, AAs respond well, along with older and younger adults, with a high strength of evidence.[18] Reducing sodium also significantly lowers BP across a wide range of patients.[19]

Reducing sodium intake in adults who eat either a typical American diet or the DASH dietary plan seems to assist with BP control with a high level of evidence. There is also a recommendation to lower sodium intake (class 1A) and to consume no more than 2400 mg of sodium per day with benefits with further reductions of sodium intake to 1500 mg of sodium per day, resulting in even greater BP reduction. Even without achieving these goals, reducing sodium intake to at least 1000 mg per day lowers BP.[19]

Potassium may be an important component of BP control. However, the potassium dietary recommendations give a low strength of evidence with insufficient evidence to determine whether increasing dietary potassium intake lowers BP, despite observational studies that link higher dietary potassium intake with lower stroke risk.[19]

Therefore, adults would benefit from lower BP by combining the DASH dietary eating plan with low sodium intake (class 1A). Additional physical activity may have a benefit (class 2A, level A). Engaging in aerobic physical activity lowered BP when performing at least 3 to 4 sessions per

Table 2
Recommendations based on the evidence available in the Joint National Committee 7 gives general support to the use of therapeutic lifestyle interventions

Modification	Recommendation	Approximate SBP Reduction (Range)
Weight reduction	Maintain normal body weight (BMI 18.5–24.9 kg/m^2).	5–20 mm Hg/10 kg
Adopt DASH eating plan	Consume a diet rich in fruits, vegetables, and low-fat dairy products with a reduced content of saturated and total fat.	8–14 mm Hg
Dietary sodium reduction	Reduce dietary sodium intake to no more than 100 mmol/d (2.4 g sodium or 6 g sodium chloride).	2–8 mm Hg
Physical activity	Engage in regular aerobic physical activity, such as brisk walking (at least 30 min/d, most days of the week).	4–9 mm Hg
Moderation of alcohol consumption	Limit consumption to no more than 2 drinks (eg, 24-oz beer, 10-oz wine, or 3-oz 80-proof whiskey) per day in most men and no more than 1 drink per day in women and lighter-weight persons.	2–4 mm Hg

From National High Blood Pressure Education Program. The seventh report of the Joint National Committee on prevention, detection, evaluation, and treatment of high blood pressure, 2004. Available at: http://www.ncbi.nlm.nih.gov/books/NBK9630/. Accessed June 5, 2016.

week, lasting an average of 40 minutes per session, involving moderate- to vigorous-intensity physical activity.[19]

PREFERRED ANTIHYPERTENSIVE PHARMACOTHERAPY: INITIAL MONOTHERAPY AND COMBINATION THERAPY

For the control of hypertension in clinical practice (**Fig. 3**), the major options for initial drug therapy without any compelling indications (ie, DM, congestive HF [CHF], CKD, MI) are as follows:

- Thiazide-type diuretics
- CCBs
- ACEis/ARBs
- Beta-blockers, limited for initial therapy in the absence of a compelling indication

CONSIDERATION OF INITIAL COMBINATION THERAPY

Each of these major 3 classes for initial antihypertensive agents is similarly effective in lowering the BP in the general adult population with an adequate antihypertensive response for stage 1 hypertension in 30% to 50% of patients (**Table 3**). Nevertheless, there remains wide interpatient variability in BP lowering across the classes in any given patient. Initial monotherapy is unlikely to attain goal BP in patients whose BPs are more than 20/10 mm Hg greater than the goal, for example, 160/100 mm

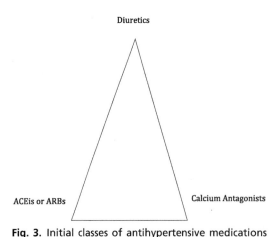

Fig. 3. Initial classes of antihypertensive medications for first step and combination therapy. Compelling indications, in general, are comorbid diseases that require certain antihypertensive drug classes for high-risk conditions. The drug selections for compelling indications are based on favorable outcome data from clinical trials, such as for reduced ejection fraction HF, post-MI, and CKD. Compelling indications may modify this.

Hg or greater. Hence, in most patients with stage 2 hypertension, and also many with stage 1 hypertension, combination therapy using 2 drugs is needed. In many cases, black patients and older patients representing low-renin hypertension types generally have a better antihypertensive effect with initial monotherapy with a thiazide-type diuretic or CCB as compared with an ACEi, ARB, or beta-blocker, if no other compelling indications exist. There is a more robust reduction in BP with diuretics and CCBs overall, as they are less sensitive to sodium intake.[20,21]

Current guidelines support using a combination as a first step with higher BP levels. This strategy may increase the likelihood that target BPs are achieved in a shorter time period, requiring fewer clinic visits and drug changes. Clinicians may consider it appropriate to use available fixed-dose combination preparations. Prescribing 2 or more drugs in a single pill may improve patient compliance, BP control, and, if both drugs are given at lower doses, reduce side effects.

Recommended combinations often include a thiazide-type diuretic or CCB added to an ACEi or ARB as first step in high-risk patients, especially with stage 2 hypertension. In the Avoiding Cardiovascular Events through Combination Therapy in Patients Living with Systolic Hypertension (ACCOMPLISH) trial, the combination of benazepril plus amlodipine was shown to be more effective than benazepril plus hydrochlorothiazide (HCTZ) in reducing CV events. Considering similar, 24-hour BP control in both treatment arms, the difference in CV outcomes favoring a renin-angiotensin system (RAS) blocker combined with amlodipine rather than HCTZ may have been impacted by differences in the intrinsic properties (metabolic or hemodynamic) of the two combination therapies.[22]

HYPERTENSION ETHNICITY TREATMENT AND CONTROL IN PERSONS WITH DIABETES

The treatment of patients who have DM and elevated BP has evolved from a lower BP goal of 130/80 mm Hg to consistent SBP of 140 mm Hg in most guidelines. This change is largely based on the lack of primary outcome benefit with intensive BP reduction in persons with type 2 DM in the ACCORD (Action to Control Cardiovascular Risk in Diabetes) study group, whereby with an average of 3 drugs, SBP of 119 mm Hg versus standard treatment to 133 mm Hg in 4733 patients showed no benefit in the primary outcome of nonfatal MI, nonfatal stroke, or CV death. Nevertheless, there was a secondary outcome, although the events were small, of nonfatal stroke and total stroke in ACCORD.[23]

Table 3
Major options for initial drug therapy in hypertension treatment

Treatment	Description
Thiazide-type diuretics	• Useful first-line agents in hypertension treatment • Proven to reduce CV morbidity and mortality • Low cost • As effective and superior to other classes • Can be successfully combined with beta-blockers, ACEis, ARBs, centrally acting agents, and CCBs
CCBs	• Dilate arteries by reducing calcium flux into cells • Effectively lowers BP across all patient groups, regardless of sex, race/ethnicity, age, and dietary sodium intake • Initial calcium antagonist can prevent all major types of CVD, except HF
ACEis	• Block the conversion of the vasoconstrictor peptide angiotensin II from its inactive decapeptide precursor, angiotensin I while simultaneously inhibiting inactivation of the vasodilator bradykinin • Benefits patients with CKD, HF, and post-MI • Effective in combination with thiazide diuretics or CCBs • No major difference in efficacy between ACEis and ARBs
ARBs	• Block angiotensin II at its receptor site • Effective antihypertensive agents • Particularly well tolerated • Benefits in conditions, such as CKD and diabetic nephropathy, chronic HF or HF following MI, and hypertension with LVH • Effective in combination with thiazide diuretics or CCBs

Data from Ferdinand KC. A compendium of antihypertensive therapy. J Clin Hypertens 2011;13(9):636–92.

Regarding the 2016 recommendations from the American Diabetes Association (ADA) for BP control in persons with DM, the ADA suggests that BP of 120/80 mm Hg should be advised for all, with lifestyle changes as needed to reduce BP. If BP is confirmed in the office as consistently greater than 140/90 mm Hg, in addition to changes in lifestyle, prompt initiation and timely subsequent titration of pharmacologic therapy to achieve BP goals are suggested with a stronger evidence level of A. Although SBP of 140 mm Hg is now consistently suggested for persons with DM as a goal, the ADA's 2016 recommendations also note that in patients who are at high risk of stroke, having a lower SBP target of less than 130 mm Hg may be beneficial, especially if it can be achieved with few drugs and without side effects. The ADA's recommendations caution lowering BPs to less than 130/70 mm Hg in older adults because of the lack of evidence in improvement of CV outcomes and the potential of higher mortality associated with treating diastolic BP (DBP) to less than 70 mm Hg. This conclusion was based on a weak level of evidence and not based on any prespecified clinical trial. The ADA also suggests a regimen that includes either an ACEi or an ARB for persons with DM, but not both. In general, the addition of 2 members of the renin-angiotensin blocking system, ACEis and ARBs together, is no longer suggested as a primary approach to persons with essential hypertension.[24]

PROTOCOL-BASED TREATMENT OF ESSENTIAL HYPERTENSION

The use of standardized treatment protocols, endorsed by the Million Hearts Program, the Veterans Administration (VA), Kaiser Permanente, and other organizations, builds on the positive experiences in BP control and the reduction in disparate outcomes.[25]

The utilization of standardized treatment protocols is now considered an effective approach to hypertension to improve BP control. Multiple protocols promulgated help clarify titration intervals, including evidence-based therapies and treatment options. Most protocols support team-based approaches and include nonphysician staff as important components of the care team, such as nurse practitioners, physician assistants, clinical assistants, and pharmacists, who can assist in timely follow-up with patients.

The VA/Department of Defense protocol focuses on the critical decision points in the management of hypertension in primary care. The protocol proposes the use of thiazide diuretics as first-line therapy and recommendations for prehypertension and treatment by stage of hypertension, along with target goals depending on patients' comorbidities (eg, DM, CKD).

The Kaiser Permanente protocol was developed for use by integrated health care delivery systems and was adopted by the 2013 ACC/AHA/Centers for Disease Control and Prevention (CDC) science report on hypertension control. The Kaiser Permanente Protocol proposes thiazide-type diuretic/ACEi combinations as first-line therapy. Moreover, when feasible, single-pill combination tablets are preferred with recommended drugs and dosages (**Fig. 4**).

The Kaiser Permanente hypertension treatment algorithm has contributed to the achievement of control rates of greater than 85% for more than 1 million US adults with hypertension. Across all ages, races, ethnicities, and both sexes, hypertension control exceeded the national average. The large Hispanic population, 39% of the population, also had 85% control, similar to that of other groups. Asians and Pacific Islanders (9% of the cohort) had 87.9% BP control.[25] Importantly, blacks, who are 8% of the cohort, had 81.4% BP control compared with 86.6% control in non-Hispanic whites (26% of the cohort). The foundation of the protocol is

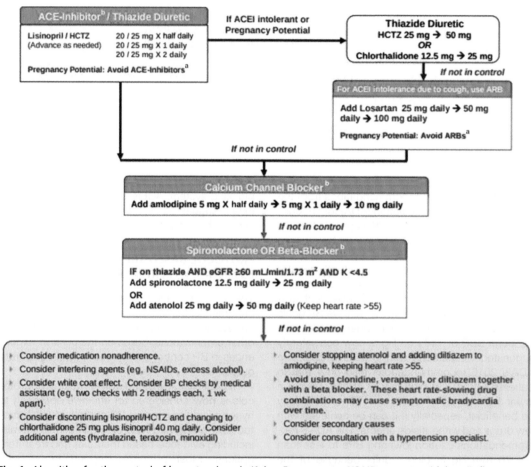

Fig. 4. Algorithm for the control of hypertension via Kaiser Permanente. NSAIDs, nonsteroidal antiinflammatory drugs. [a] CKD is defined as albuminuria (>30 mg of albumin/g of creatinine) at any age and any level of GFR, or an estimated GFR or measured GFR <60 mL/min/1.73 m^2, antihypertensive treatment should be individualized, taking into consideration factors such as frailty, comorbidities, albuminuria, and estimation of non-age-related eGFR decline (eg, if eGFR + 1/2 age is <85). [b] ACE-inhibitors and ARBs are contraindicated in pregnancy and not recommended in most women of childbearing age. Calcium Channel Blockers and Spironolactone (Pregnancy Risk Category C), and Beta-Blockers (Pregnancy Risk Category D) should only be used in pregnancy when clearly needed and the benefits outweigh the potential hazard to the fetus. (*From* Kaiser Permanente Care Management Institute. Management of adult hypertension. In: KP national hypertension guideline - clinician guide, 2014. Available at: http://kpcmi.org/files/kp-hypertension-algorithm.pdf. Accessed June 5, 2016; with permission.)

the fixed-dose combination drug lisinopril/HCTZ, maximized in 3 steps before adding amlodipine. As confirmed by increasing antihypertensive clinical trial evidence, spironolactone is the preferred fourth drug.[26]

Salient Kaiser Permanente that can be adopted by other systems and practitioners include among other aspects

- Team-based care
- Convenient BP checks
- Population registry
- Quality performance goals
- Quality performance tracking metrics
- Self-monitoring BP

Overall, protocols and systems-based approaches may lead to more comprehensive hypertension control if adopted in a more widespread manner. Although protocols can be modified for adoption and use, health care professionals should always consider the patients' individual clinical circumstances.

The following is a summary of principles recommended for creating an effective hypertension management algorithm:

- Base algorithm components and processes on the best available science.
- The format should be simple to update as better information becomes available.
- Create a feasible, simple implementation strategy.
- Include the patient version at an appropriate scientific and language literacy level.
- Consider costs of diagnosis, monitoring, and treatment.
- Develop an algorithm in a format easily used within a team approach to health care.
- Develop an algorithm in a format that can be incorporated into electronic health records for use as clinical decision support.
- Include a disclaimer to ensure that the algorithm is not used to counter the treating health care provider's best clinical judgment.[15]

There are several steps clinicians can use when approaching patients with hypertension. In view of the dismal rates of adherence, it is important to include patient understanding by

- Limiting the amount of information provided at each visit
- Slowing down
- Avoiding medical jargon
- Using pictures or models to explain important concepts

- Assuring understanding with the show-me technique
- Encouraging patients to ask questions[15,26,27]

Recent Guidelines and Reports of Treatment of Hypertension

The expert treatment of essential hypertension requires individual assessment and choices. Nevertheless, multiple contemporary guidelines direct clinical practice and goal attainment. Recent hypertension guidelines and reports with recommendations for BP goals and targets as well as providing important pathways for effective BP control and decreasing CV outcomes have included the following:

- The 2013 European Society of Hypertension (ESH)/European Society of Cardiology (ESC) guidelines for the management of arterial hypertension: the Task Force for the Management of Arterial Hypertension of the ESH and of the ESC[28]
- Clinical practice guidelines for the management of hypertension in the community: a statement by the American Society of Hypertension (ASH) and the International Society of Hypertension (ISH)[29]
- An effective approach to high BP control: a science advisory from the AHA, ACC, and CDC[18]
- 2014 Evidence-Based Guideline for the Management of High Blood Pressure in Adults: Report from the Panel Members Appointed to the Eighth Joint National Committee (JNC 8)[30]

In addition, the ADA's practice recommendations give practical suggestions on the management of BP in persons with DM.[24]

Overall, these guidelines and reports provide consistency in that initiation of drug therapy with 2 drugs is suggested in patients with markedly elevated BP or stage 2 hypertension (BP $\geq$160/100 mm Hg) (**Table 4**). Additionally, BP targets are noted as less than 140/90 mm Hg for most patients with hypertension. There are various approaches to the consideration of higher targets in elderly patients who are 80 years of age and greater. The ESH/ESC's guidelines suggest SBP of 140 to 150 in elderly patients, whereas the ASH/ISH's recommendations suggest BP of less than 150/90.[28,29] The 2014 US hypertension guidelines, published by members originally appointed to the JNC 8, are somewhat unique in that for patients as young as 60 years or older, a goal of less than 150/90 mm Hg is recommended.[30]

Table 4
Blood pressure targets (mm Hg) based on recent hypertension guidelines and reports

	ESH/ESC 2013	ASH/ISH 2014	Go et al AHA/ACC/CDC 2013	Hypertension Guidelines, US JNC 8 2014
Initiate drug therapy with 2 drugs	In patients with markedly elevated BP	≥160/100 mm Hg	≥160/100 mm Hg	≥160/100 mm Hg
BP targets	<140/90 mm Hg Elderly <80 y SBP 140–150 mm Hg SBP <140 mm Hg in fit patients Elderly ≥80 y SBP 140–150 mm Hg	<140/90 mm Hg Elderly ≥80 y BP <150/90	<140/90 mm Hg Lower targets may be appropriate in some, including the elderly	<60 y BP <140/90 mm Hg >60 y BP <150/90 mm Hg
BP targets in patients with DM	<140/85 mm Hg	<140/90 mm Hg	<140/90 mm Hg Lower targets may be considered	<140/90 mm Hg

Data from Refs.[15,18,28–30]

BP targets for persons with DM have consistently now suggested less than 140 mm Hg SBP with DBP of 85 mm Hg and 90 mm Hg in different reports.[18] The ADA's 2016 recommendations also support less than 140/90 mm Hg as compared with the previous less than 130/80 mm Hg. The AHA/ACC/CDC's report, however, suggested 140/90 mm Hg for all persons, including the elderly, and suggested even lower targets may be appropriate in some patients, including those with DM.[24]

The AHA/ACC/CDC's report was not a full evidence-based guideline but rather a science advisory that suggested effective approaches for high BP control. It gave an algorithm seeking to lower BP to less than 140/90 for all adults with hypertension and suggested the combination approach with an ACEi and thiazide diuretic as a first step with additional CCB, spironolactone, and beta-blockers as needed. To a large extent, the AHA/ACC/CDC's science advisory reproduces the algorithm used at Kaiser Permanente, an integrated health care delivery system, which has demonstrated excellent BP control across all populations regardless of race and ethnicity.[18]

2014 EVIDENCE-BASED GUIDELINES FOR THE MANAGEMENT OF HIGH BLOOD PRESSURE IN ADULTS

The *2014 Evidence-Based Guidelines for the Management of High Blood Pressure in Adults* was not an approved National Heart Lung and Blood Institute guideline article. Although the

report was from panel members originally appointed to JNC 8, the US 2014 guideline was based on a rigorous review of present evidence of randomized trials with greater than 100 patients and hard CV outcomes.[30]

Their algorithm suggests the use of thiazide diuretics, ACEis or ARBs or CCB alone or in combination in most patients. However, specifically for black patients, initiating thiazide-type diuretic or CCB alone or in combination was recommended, if there are no compelling indications for the use of the other antihypertensive agents. For persons of all races with CKD, initiation with ACEi or ARB alone or in combination with other drug classes was suggested (**Fig. 5**).[30]

Nevertheless, despite the rigorous evidence used in the development of the 2014 US guidelines, various published reports have taken issue with their suggestion of a lower goal of less than 150/90 mm Hg for persons who are 60 years of age and younger.[31] One state-of-the-art review suggested that increasing the elderly goal to less than 150/90 mm Hg would be inappropriate and potentially do harm, especially to elderly, black, and female patients. The view of the investigators was that a new BP goal of less than 150/90 mm Hg would specifically affect these populations who are at higher risk, because there are more elderly women with hypertension, and AAs that have an increased risk of morbidity and mortality related to elevated BP. Notably, hypertension-related death rates in non-Hispanic blacks approximately doubles that seen in Hispanics and non-Hispanic whites.[32]

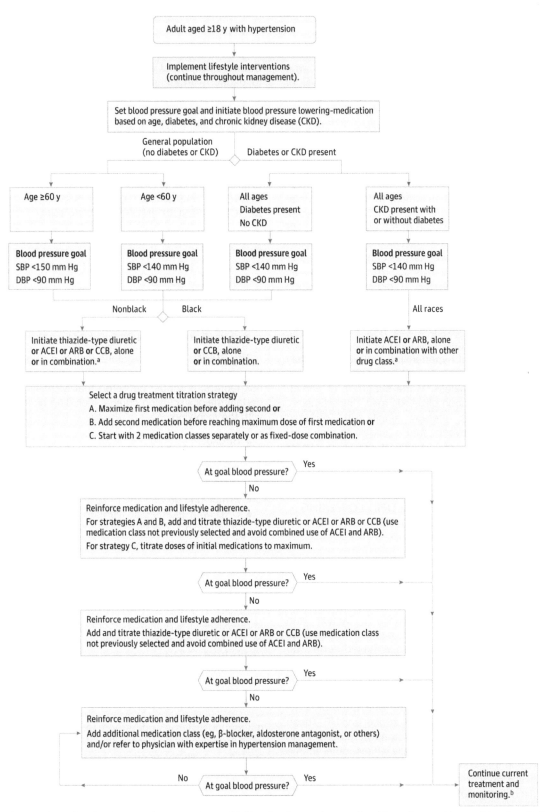

Fig. 5. Algorithm for 2014 US hypertension guideline. [a] ACEIs and ARBs should not be used in combination. [b] If blood pressure fails to be maintained at goal, reenter the algorithm where appropriate based on the current individual therapeutic plan. (*From* James PA, Oparil S, Carter BL, et al. 2014 Evidence-based guideline for the management of high blood pressure in adults: report from the panel members appointed to the eighth joint national committee (JNC 8). JAMA 2014;311(5):516; with permission.)

Hypertension guidelines have recommended the addition of spironolactone to patients who are on triple drug therapy with a diuretic, CCB, or RAS-blocking agent. Recent evidence from the Prevention And Treatment of Hypertension With Algorithm-based therapy trial demonstrated the superiority of spironolactone versus placebo, bisoprolol and doxazosin as an add-on treatment of drug-resistant hypertension.[33]

In the recent Heart Outcomes Prevention Evaluation (HOPE-3) trial, treatment with candesartan at a dosage of 16 mg/d plus HCTZ at a dosage of 12.5 mg/d over a period of 5.6 years lowered BP by 6.0/3.0 mm Hg from baseline but did not result in a significantly lower risk, as compared with placebo, of major CV events. The cohort was an intermediate-risk versus a high-risk population without CVD and with very low rates of DM (5.8%) and mild renal dysfunction (2.8%). The average BP at baseline was 138.1/81.9 mm Hg, with approximately one-third of the participants with a history of hypertension and approximately 22% of participants taking antihypertensive agents. Nevertheless, in the subgroup of participants with uncomplicated mild hypertension, antihypertensive therapy significantly reduced the risk of CV events; future guidelines may suggest a benefit of pharmacotherapy in similar cohorts.[34]

TREATMENT LESSONS LEARNED FROM THE ANTIHYPERTENSIVE AND LIPID LOWERING TREATMENT TO PREVENT HEART ATTACK TRIAL

After lifestyle modification, particularly diet and physical activity, most evidence-based guidelines now suggest diuretics, calcium antagonists, ACEis, or ARBs as first-step agents, whereas the 2014 US guidelines specifically indicate a benefit with thiazide-type diuretics and calcium antagonists for blacks.[30] This indication is based largely on the outcomes from the ALLHAT trial, the largest antihypertensive study ever completed. Compared with lisinopril, those patients who are defined as black on chlorthalidone had lower rates of combined CHD, combined CVD, stroke, and HF. These types of differences in outcomes were not seen in nonblack patients, essentially whites, other than a small increase in combined CVD and a small trend toward an increase in HF. Primarily as a consequence of the outcomes of ALLHAT, chlorthalidone was found to be the most effective approach as initial therapy in high-risk patients with hypertension, with the effect being most pronounced in the black subgroup. Interestingly, the risk of ESRD was not reduced by lisinopril compared with

chlorthalidone in either subgroup, although the CIs were somewhat wide.[35] Another consideration for caution with using ACEi in blacks may be related to the increased risk of angioedema developed related to regional vasodilatation and increased vascular permeability that can occur even long-term after the use of ACEis. This increase is another risk more prominent in blacks.[36]

TREATMENT OF HYPERTENSION IN OLDER PERSONS: THE IMPACT OF THE SYSTOLIC BLOOD PRESSURE INTERVENTION TRIAL

Future guidelines and working group reports will be influenced by the results of the SPRINT trial. This large National Institutes of Health study recruited 9361 patients:

- 38% of whom are black and minorities
- 30% of whom are aged 75 years or older
- 20% of whom had previous CVD[37]

The SPRINT inclusion criteria included persons 50 years or older with hypertension and additional risk factors. It should be noted that SPRINT had certain major exclusion criteria, including persons with the following:

- Stroke
- DM
- Polycystic kidney disease
- CHF (symptoms or ejection fraction <35%)
- Proteinuria greater than 1 g/d
- CKD with glomerular filtration rate less than 20 mL/min/1.73 m^2
- Adherence concerns

The SPRINT investigators should be congratulated as they were able to achieve significant BP lowering in the intensive arm to 121.5 mm Hg, as opposed to 134.6 mm Hg in the standard arm. Impressively, the primary outcome of a composite of MI, acute coronary syndrome, stroke, HF, or death from CVD was positive. Death from any cause was also positive.[37]

Subgroup analyses of SPRINT suggest that other than persons with DM, HF, or severe CKD, SPRINT can be widely applied. However, the number of females studied largely underrepresented the burden of hypertension in that population. This underrepresentation possibly occurred because of higher recruitment from the predominantly male VA medical centers. Nevertheless, SPRINT seemed to be beneficial in the following populations:

- Patients with or without previous CKD
- Patients aged 75 years or older
- Male and female patients
- Black and nonblack patients

- Patients having previous CVD or not
- Patients having various levels of entry SBP, including significant lowering with pressures of 132 mm Hg at baseline

Among 2636 participants (mean age, 79.9 years; 37.9% women), there was a significantly lower rate of the primary composite outcome (102 events in the intensive treatment group vs 148 events in the standard treatment group; hazard ratio [HR], 0.66 [95% CI, 0.51–0.85]) and all-cause mortality (73 deaths vs 107 deaths, respectively; HR, 0.67 [95% CI, 0.49–0.91]).[37]

The overall rate of serious adverse events was not different between treatment groups (48.4% in the intensive treatment group vs 48.3% in the standard treatment group; HR, 0.99 [95% CI, 0.89–1.11]); there was no significant increase in absolute rates of hypotension, syncope, electrolyte abnormalities, or acute kidney injury. The investigators concluded that among ambulatory adults aged 75 years and older, treating to an SBP target of less than 120 mm Hg compared with an SBP target of less than 140 mm Hg resulted in significantly lower rates of fatal and nonfatal major CV events and death from any cause.[37] These data add to evidence supporting more intensive BP goals, even in persons older than 75 years.[18]

Comparing Systolic Blood Pressure Intervention Trial and ACCORD

One question that arose regards the important differences between SPRINT and ACCORD.

- The SPRINT cohort was older, with a mean age of 68 years as compared with 62 years for ACCORD.
- The SPRINT cohort included patients with CKD.
- The sample size of ACCORD (4773) was approximately half that of SPRINT (9661).

The SPRINT investigators suggested that the difference in results could be due to differences in study design, treatment interaction, or play of chance. However, investigators question the inherent differences in CV benefits of SBP lowering between populations of patients with or without DM. An important component of the SPRINT trial was the ability to successfully lower BP in high-risk patients who are middle aged and older.[18,37,38]

SUGGESTED ANTIHYPERTENSIVE AGENTS FOR EFFECTIVE BLOOD PRESSURE CONTROL IN SYSTOLIC BLOOD PRESSURE INTERVENTION TRIAL

Although not a specific drug comparison trial, certain recommendations were made for the SPRINT trial investigators to optimize BP control that can be applied in clinical medicine. These suggested practices for BP lowering are shown in **Table 5**.

ADVANCES IN HYPERTENSION CONTROL: PATIENT-CENTERED CARE

The treatment of essential hypertension has now moved beyond the conventional physician clinic

Table 5
Recommendations made by Systolic Blood Pressure Intervention Trial investigators

Chlorthalidone (12.5–25.0 mg/d) thiazide-type diuretic of choice	Recommended More potent and longer acting than hydrochlorothiazide
Amlodipine CCB (of choice)	Recommended
ACEis (and likely other RAS blockers)	Less effective compared with other classes in lowering BP and preventing CVD events in AAs, unless combined with a thiazide-type diuretic or CCB
Loop diuretic (eg, furosemide)	May be needed with advanced CKD (eGFR <30 mL/min/1.73m²)
Any combination of ACEi, ARB, and renin inhibitor	Discouraged
Beta-blockers	Less effective in preventing CVD events as primary hypertension treatment but may be needed with CAD
Minoxidil	Diuretic also recommended with use
α2-agonist guanfacine (1–3 mg/d) or clonidine skin patch vs oral clonidine	Recommended because of longer duration of action allowing daily guanfacine or weekly clonidine patch

From Eckel RH, Jakicic JM, Ard JD, et al. 2013 AHA/ACC guideline on lifestyle management to reduce cardiovascular risk: a report of the American College of Cardiology/American Heart Association Task Force on Practice Guidelines. J Am Coll Cardiol 2014;63(25_PA); with permission.

visit; BP control now includes self-monitoring of BP, as recommended by the Community Preventive Services Task Force and others.[39] The Million Hearts Campaign (http://millionhearts.hhs.gov/) is a national initiative of the Department of Health and Human Services whose goal is to prevent 1 million heart attacks and strokes by 2017. This collaborative effort involves multiple government agencies and nongovernmental collaborators; one of its main areas of focus is improving medication adherence through knowledge dissemination, stakeholder activation, creation of incentives, measuring and reporting, improving population health, and research. Million Hearts has also suggested that BP improves when care is provided by a team of health care professionals rather than a single physician. This shift may increase the proportion of patients with controlled BP, decrease SBP and DBP, and improve patient outcomes not only for BP but also for DM and blood lipids.[40]

Home BP monitoring is an additional measure widely accepted to improve BP control along with team-based care for optimal care. Efforts to control BP, especially in blacks, older women, and high-risk patients, should continue to focus on the increasing the number of patients who have BPs controlled to less than 140/90 mm Hg, with perhaps even more intensive therapy based on the SPRINT trial.[37] Multidrug regimens in higher-risk patients include adequate diuretic, especially chlorthalidone, RAS-blocking agents, ACEis, ARBs, and long-acting CCBs. In resistant hypertension, spironolactone will be considered an additionally effective approach.

Therapeutic lifestyle changes are essential for BP control in addition to pharmacotherapy. Recently, the US Food and Drug Administration (FDA) released a 2016 draft guidance for public comment that provides voluntary sodium reduction targets for the food industry. The FDA proposes to decrease in the short-term sodium intake to about 3000 mg/d; long-term (10-year) targets seek to reduce sodium intake to 2300 mg/d, linking diets high in sodium to hypertension and as a major risk factor for heart disease and stroke. Because 70% of sodium comes in the form of processed and prepared food, the FDA seeks to complement many existing efforts by food manufacturers, restaurants, and food service operations to reduce sodium in foods.[41] In addition, the most recent US dietary guidelines recommend limiting intake of sodium to less than 2300 mg/d for individuals aged 14 years or older, supporting the benefits a population-based approach to decreasing hypertension prevalence.[42]

EMERGING AND FUTURE GUIDELINES IN THE TREATMENT OF ESSENTIAL HYPERTENSION

UpToDate is an evidence-based clinical decision support resource designed to assist health care practitioners to help them make correct, contemporary decisions at the point of care and improve outcomes. Their following recommendation for goal BP is for patients with increased risk of a CV event defined as aged 75 years or older, clinically evident CVD (ie, previously documented coronary, peripheral arterial, or cerebrovascular disease [except for stroke]), subclinical CVD (ie, an elevated coronary artery calcification score by computerized tomography scan, LVH, or an ankle-brachial index <0.9), an eGFR of 20 to 59 mL/min/1.73 m^2, or a 10-year Framingham Risk Score of 15% or greater.[5]

In 2016, their experts recommended in high-risk patients targeting a BP of 120 to 125/less than 90 mm Hg rather than less than 140/90 mm Hg if AOBP measurements are used rather than a higher goal BP (grade 1A).[5]

If conventional clinic measurements are obtained, it is recommended to target a BP of 125 to 130/less than 90 mm Hg rather than less than 140/90 mm Hg. In patients with DM, a BP goal of 120 to 125/less than 90 mm Hg (if AOBP readings are used) or 125 to 130/less than 90 mm Hg (if manual auscultatory measurements are used) rather than a goal BP of less than 140/less than 90 mm Hg (using manual auscultatory measurements) is recommended (grade 2B).

The recommendations for persons with DM are based on data from various goal BP trials in diabetic patients, plus indirect data from the high-risk nondiabetic SPRINT. Future evidence-based major guidelines may similarly recommend a range of BP levels as goals with more intensive BP lowering and goals for patients with and without DM.

The ACC/AHA's pending guidelines on the management of hypertension are expected to recommend more intensive therapy versus less intensive therapy for the control of BP across multiple populations.[43]

SUMMARY

Hypertension and CVD are highly prevalent in the United States and a main cause of death. Hypertension prevalence, control, and outcomes display disparities by race and ethnicity, which are sizable, likely multifactorial, and to a large extent preventable. CVD related to hypertension, specifically HF, ESRD, CAD events, and stroke, diminish longevity in blacks. These disparities are primarily due to a combination of social determinants of health, risk factor control, culture, and environment. The 3 major classes for initial therapy for adults with hypertension are thiazide-type diuretics, CCBs, and ACEi/ARBs, with diuretics and CCBs preferred in most blacks as the first step, unless compelling indications are noted. Hypertension is controlled by therapeutic lifestyle changes, especially weight loss and sodium restriction; but most patients require pharmacotherapy, often with 2 or more drugs in combination. Those patients at highest risk benefit from more intensive intervention. Potentially, effective hypertension treatment protocols and team-based care, combined with home BP monitoring, will significantly reduce the unacceptable high levels of uncontrolled hypertension in all patients.

REFERENCES

1. O'Donnell AJ, Bogner HR, Kellom K, et al. Stakeholder perspectives on changes in hypertension care under the patient-centered medical home. Prev Chronic Dis 2016;13:E28.
2. WHO. A global brief on hypertension, 2013. Available at: http://ish-world.com/downloads/pdf/global_brief_hypertension.pdf. Accessed June 5, 2016.
3. Ettehad D, Emdin CA, Kiran A, et al. Blood pressure lowering for prevention of cardiovascular disease and death: a systematic review and meta-analysis. Lancet 2016;387(10022):957–67.
4. National High Blood Pressure Education Program. The seventh report of the Joint National Committee on Prevention, Detection, Evaluation, and Treatment of High Blood Pressure, 2004. Available at: http://www.ncbi.nlm.nih.gov/books/NBK9630/. Accessed June 5, 2016.
5. Bakris GL, White WB, et al. Goal blood pressure in patients with cardiovascular disease or at high risk. Available at: http://www.uptodate.com/contents/goal-blood-pressure-in-patients-with-cardiovascular-disease-or-at-high-risk?source=related_link. Accessed June 19, 2016.
6. Kieldsen SE, Lund-Johansen P, Nilsson PM, et al. Unattended blood pressure measurements in the Systolic Blood Pressure Intervention Trial: implications for entry and achieved blood pressure values compared with other trials. Hypertension 2016; 67(5):808–12.
7. Egan BM, Zhao Y, Axon RN, et al. US trends in prevalence, awareness, treatment, and control of hypertension, 1988-2008. JAMA 2010;303(20): 2043–50.
8. Yoon SS, et al. NCHS data brief, no 220. In: National Center for Health Statistics, 2015. Available at: http://www.cdc.gov/nchs/products/databriefs/db220.htm. Accessed June 5, 2016.
9. Flack JM, Sica DA, Bakris G, et al, for the International Society on Hypertension in Blacks. Management of high blood pressure in blacks: an update of the International Society on Hypertension in Blacks consensus statement. Hypertension 2010; 56:780–800.
10. Frieden ET. CDC health disparities and inequalities report — United States, 2011. MMWR Suppl 2011; 60(1):1–112.
11. Ferdinand KC, Ferdinand DP. Race-based therapy for hypertension: possible benefits and potential pitfalls. Expert Rev Cardiovasc Ther 2008;10:1357–66.
12. USRDS. Incidence, prevalence, patient characteristics and modality. In: 2012 Atlas of end-stage renal disease. Available at: http://www.usrds.org/2012/pdf/v2_ch1_12.pdf. Accessed June 5, 2016.
13. Schieb LJ, Greer SA, Ritchey MD, et al. Vital signs: avoidable deaths from heart disease, stroke, and hypertensive disease — United States, 2001–2010. MMWR 2013;62(35):721–7.
14. Kochanek KD, et al. Deaths: final data for 2009. In: Center for Health Statistics, 2011; Available at: http://www.cdc.gov/nchs/data/nvsr/nvsr60/nvsr60_03.pdf. Accessed June 5, 2016.
15. Go AS, Bauman MA, Coleman King SM, et al. An effective approach to high blood pressure control: a science advisory from the American Heart Association, the American College of Cardiology, and the Centers for Disease Control and Prevention. J Am Coll Cardiol 2014;63(12): 1230–8.
16. Nesbitt SD. Hypertension in black patients: special issues and considerations. Curr Hypertens Rep 2005;7:244–8.
17. Goutham R, Powell-Wiley TM, Ancheta I, et al. Identification of obesity and cardiovascular risk in ethnically and racially diverse populations: a scientific statement from the American Heart Association. Circulation 2015;132(5):457–72.
18. Eckel RH, Jakicic JM, Ard JD, et al. 2013 AHA/ACC guideline on lifestyle management to reduce cardiovascular risk: a report of the American College of Cardiology/American Heart Association Task Force on Practice Guidelines. J Am Coll Cardiol 2014; 129(25 Suppl 2):S76–99.
19. Mozaffarian D, Benjamin EJ, Go AS, et al. Heart disease and stroke statistics - 2015 update: a report from the American Heart Association. Circulation 2015;131:e29–322.
20. Gadegbeku CA, Lea JP, Jamerson KA. Update on disparities in the pathophysiology and management of hypertension: focus on African Americans. Med Clin North Am 2005;89:921–33, 930.
21. Flack JM, Sica DA. Therapeutic considerations in the African-American patient with hypertension: considerations with calcium channel blocker therapy 2005;7(4 Suppl 1):9–14.

22. Jamerson K, Weber MA, Bakris GL, et al, for the ACCOMPLISH Trial Investigators. Benazepril plus amlodipine or hydrochlorothiazide for hypertension in high-risk patients. N Engl J Med 2008;359:2417–28.

23. The ACCORD Study Group. Effects of combination lipid therapy in type 2 diabetes mellitus. N Engl J Med 2010;362:1563–74.

24. American Diabetes Association. Standards of Medical Care in Diabetes. Diabetes Care 2016; 39(Suppl 1):S60–71.

25. Shaw KM, Handler J, Wall HK, et al. Improving blood pressure control in a large multiethnic California population through changes in health care delivery, 2004–2012. Prev Chronic Dis 2014;11:140173.

26. Handler J. Commentary in support of a highly effective hypertension treatment algorithm. J Clin Hypertens 2013;15:874–7.

27. Weiss BD. Health literacy and patient safety: help patients understand. Manual for clinicians, 2nd edition. In: Health literacy educational toolkit, 2nd edition, 2007. Available at: http://www.ama-assn.org/resources/doc/ama-foundation/x-pub/healthlitclinicians.pdf. Accessed June 5, 2016.

28. Mancia G, Fagard R, Narkiewicz K, et al. 2013 ESH/ESC guidelines for the management of arterial hypertension: the Task Force for the Management of Arterial Hypertension of the European Society of Hypertension (ESH) and of the European Society of Cardiology (ESC). J Hypertens 2013;31(7):1281–357.

29. Weber MA, Schiffrin EL, White WB, et al. Clinical practice guidelines for the management of hypertension in the community: a statement by the American Society of Hypertension and the International Society of Hypertension. J Clin Hypertens 2014; 16(1):14–26.

30. James PA, Oparil S, Carter BL, et al. 2014 evidence-based guideline for the management of high blood pressure in adults: report from the panel members appointed to the Eighth Joint National Committee (JNC 8). JAMA 2014;311(5):507–20.

31. Krakoff LR, Gillespie RL, Ferdinand KC, et al. 2014 hypertension recommendations from the Eighth Joint National Committee panel members raise concerns for elderly black and female populations. J Am Coll Cardiol 2014;64:394–402.

32. Kung HC, Xu JQ. Hypertension-related mortality in the United States, 2000–2013. NCHS Data Brief 2015;(193):1–8. Available at: http://www.cdc.gov/nchs/data/databriefs/db193.pdf. Accessed June 2, 2016.

33. Williams B, MacDonald TM, Morant S, et al. Spironolactone versus placebo, bisoprolol, and doxazosin to determine the optimal treatment for drug-resistant hypertension (PATHWAY-2): a randomised, double-blind, crossover trial. Lancet 2015;386:2059–68.

34. Lonn EM, Bosch J, López-Jaramillo P, et al. Blood-pressure lowering in intermediate-risk persons without cardiovascular disease. N Engl J Med 2016;374:2009–20.

35. Wright JT, Dunn JK, Cutler JA, et al. Outcomes in hypertensive black and nonblack patients treated with chlorthalidone, amlodipine, and lisinopril. JAMA 2005;293:1595–608.

36. Bramante RM, Rand M. Images in clinical medicine. Angioedema. N Engl J Med 2011;365:e4.

37. SPRINT Research Group, Wright JT Jr, Williamson JD, et al. A randomized trial of intensive versus standard blood-pressure control. N Engl J Med 2015;373(22):2103–16.

38. Percovic V, Rodgers A. Redefining blood-pressure targets — SPRINT starts the marathon. N Engl J Med 2015;373:2175–8.

39. Cardiovascular disease prevention and control: clinical decision-support systems (CDSS). In: the guide to community preventive services, 2015. Available at: http://www.thecommunityguide.org/cvd/CDSS.html. Accessed June 16, 2016.

40. Centers for Disease Control and Prevention. Undiagnosed hypertension. Available at: http://millionhearts.hhs.gov/tools-protocols/hiding-plain-sight/index.html. Accessed June 5, 2016.

41. Food and Drug Administration. Constituent update. In: FDA issues draft guidance to industry for voluntarily reducing sodium. Available at: http://www.fda.gov/Food/NewsEvents/ConstituentUpdates/ucm504264.htm. Accessed June 1, 2016.

42. U.S. Department of Health and Human Services and U.S. Department of Agriculture. 2015 – 2020 Dietary guidelines for Americans: 8th edition, 2015. Available at: http://health.gov/dietaryguidelines/2015/guidelines. Accessed June 5, 2016.

43. Casteel B, Thacker C, et al. Hypertension guideline writing process underway. In: The AHA/ASA newsroom. Available at: http://newsroom.heart.org/news/hypertension-guideline-writing-process-underway. Accessed June 5, 2016.

Balancing Overscreening and Underdiagnosis in Secondary Hypertension
The Case of Fibromuscular Dysplasia

 CrossMark

Marcel Ruzicka, MD, PhD[a], Sarah E. Kucharski, MA[b,c],
Swapnil Hiremath, MD, MPH[a,*]

KEYWORDS

- Secondary hypertension • Renovascular hypertension • Fibromuscular dysplasia • Hypertension
- Screening • Renal artery stenosis

KEY POINTS

- The prevalence of fibromuscular dysplasia (FMD) is higher than originally thought.
- FMD affects the extrarenal vascular bed nearly as frequently as it affects the renal arteries.
- Symptoms of extrarenal FMD can be vague and nonspecific.
- Low awareness of extrarenal FMD by physicians and patients results in delayed diagnosis and missed opportunity to prevent catastrophic vascular events.
- Adverse outcomes of undiagnosed and untreated extrarenal FMD are debilitating and life threatening.

INTRODUCTION
Historical Perspective

The discovery of the role of the renal artery and hypertension dates back to the first half of the twentieth century. Experiments by Goldblatt and colleagues[1] established that narrowing of the renal artery, resulting in significant impairment of renal blood flow, induces renal renin and leads to arterial hypertension. Because treatment of severe hypertension at that time was limited principally to extreme dietary salt restriction and dorsal lumbar sympathectomy, alternative surgical treatment (in this case renal autotransplant and/or bypass of the affected renal artery) provided a reasonable treatment option for patients with renal artery stenosis. However, it became clear, even at the early stages, that not all stenoses of the renal artery were the same with regard to cause. In addition to atherosclerotic renal artery stenosis, Leadbetter and Burkland[2] in 1938 reported cure of hypertension in response to unilateral nephrectomy in a

Disclosures: M. Ruzicka and S. Hiremath receive salary support from the Department of Medicine, University of Ottawa. There was no specific funding received to support this article. S.E. Kucharski is the CEO/Chairman and Founder of FMD Chat, a nonprofit medical organization. In addition, she serves on the Rare Disease Advisory Board for Collaborations Pharmaceuticals and Morehead Planetarium's Alumni Council at the University of North Carolina–Chapel Hill. M. Ruzicka and S. Hiremath do not have any relevant financial conflicts of interest to declare.
[a] Division of Nephrology, The Ottawa Hospital, University of Ottawa, 1967 Riverside Drive, Ottawa, ON K1H7W9, Canada; [b] E-Patient Programs, Medicinex, Stanford University, 300 Pasteur Drive, Grant Building, Room S268, Stanford, CA 94305, USA; [c] FMDCHAT, Canton, NC 28716, USA
* Corresponding author.
E-mail address: shiremath@toh.ca

Cardiol Clin 35 (2017) 247–254
http://dx.doi.org/10.1016/j.ccl.2016.12.006
0733-8651/17/© 2016 Elsevier Inc. All rights reserved.

5.5-year-old boy with severe hypertension and a renal artery partially occluded by a prominent intra-arterial mass of smooth muscle. The term fibromuscular dysplasia (FMD) was first used in the setting of hypertension and renal artery stenosis by McCormack and colleagues in 1958.[3] During the following decade, FMD was recognized in extrarenal territories, including cerebrovascular (carotid and vertebral arteries), mesenteric arteries, arteries of upper and lower extremities, and coronary arteries. Harrison and McCormack[4] proposed a histologic classification of 3 distinct types of FMD based on the arterial layer most affected: intimal, medial, and adventitial/periarterial. Over the years, the most common adverse features of the natural history of FMD, such as arterial stenosis/occlusion, dissection, and aneurysm, were recognized. Clinical manifestation of these based on the part of the arterial tree involved were described. Treatment options evolved from surgical revascularization and clipping of aneurysms to catheter-based (angioplasty with/without stenting for stenosis, stents for dissections, and coils and stents for aneurysms) and medical management (antiplatelet, antithrombotic, and antihypertensive therapy, and lifestyle modification).[5]

Progress, and the Lack of It, over the Last 8 Decades

Thus, clearly, over the last several decades, major progress has been made with regard to the ability to diagnose FMD and management options to prevent catastrophic vascular outcomes. In contrast, a comprehensive review on FMD by Plouin and colleagues[6] was published as recently as in 2007 in the *Orphanet Journal of Rare Disease*, highlighting the still limited awareness of FMD by physicians and patients. In 2014, a Scientific Statement from the American Heart Association on Fibromuscular Dysplasia, published in *Circulation*, indicated that "an average delay from the time of the first symptom or sign to the diagnosis of FMD is 4 to 9 years."[7] As highlighted by the case presented later in this article, this delay or even a missed diagnosis of FMD can lead to catastrophic vascular outcomes. This article solely focuses on 2 major features crucial to the case presented later; namely the nonspecific signs and symptoms of this disease, and its prevalence in extrarenal vascular beds, which, in contrast with the older dogma of being extremely rare, is nearly equal to its occurrence in renal arteries.

Case report

A 34-year-old woman was referred to the renal hypertension clinic, from the stroke rehabilitation unit, for assessment of hypertension, specifically to consider secondary hypertension. She was recovering from a left hemiparesis, associated with a right internal carotid artery dissection, and her blood pressure in the rehabilitation unit was persistently high (>180/110 mm Hg) despite 3 antihypertensive agents. Urinary catecholamines had been done and found to be high, hence the referral was made to investigate and treat for pheochromocytoma.

She was first diagnosed to have high blood pressure when she was 30 years old, during her first (and only) pregnancy. She was started on an antihypertensive medication, but did not recall how well her blood pressure was controlled. She had been a smoker until then, and quit smoking, as well as losing 18 kg (40 pounds) over the next few months in an effort to control blood pressure. Four years after the diagnosis of hypertension, she developed transient blurring of vision and a headache one evening while jogging. The next morning, she developed left-sided hemiparesis and diplopia. Imaging revealed an acute infarct in the right middle cerebral artery (MCA) territory. A computed tomography (CT) angiogram revealed an internal carotid artery dissection, just distal to the bifurcation of the common carotid artery. There was also thrombosis seen in the proximal right MCA. Her course was complicated by cerebral edema and midline shift, requiring a craniotomy, and a subsequent deep venous thrombosis and pulmonary embolism. She required a prolonged rehabilitation stay, during which it was found that the blood pressure was not well controlled despite bisoprolol 5 mg daily, ramipril 2.5 mg daily, and hydrochlorothiazide 25 mg daily. A 24-hour urinary epinephrine was 40 nmol/d (laboratory range for normal, <100 nmol/d), norepinephrine 898 nmol/d (normal, <500), and dopamine 2708 nmol/d (normal, <2600). At the first visit to our clinic, resting blood pressure measurements, performed with an automated monitor, on the same therapy, revealed a blood pressure of 123/81 mm Hg. Serum creatinine level was 58 μmol/L and potassium level was 3.4 mmol/L. There was no proteinuria. Electrocardiogram and echocardiogram did not reveal left ventricular hypertrophy.

Because of the history of carotid dissection, a renal CT angiogram was ordered, which showed that the renal arteries were abnormal with intermittent stenotic and poststenotic ectasia, having a string-of-beads appearance in keeping with FMD. After discussion with the patient about potential benefits and risks, catheter angiogram was performed, which revealed a beaded appearance with multiple webs consistent with FMD within the terminal left renal artery and continuing throughout the length of a large upper pole branch (**Fig. 1**). A similar appearance was present involving the distal two-thirds of the right main renal artery and extending for a short distance into the large first-order branch to the upper pole. Bilateral balloon angioplasty was performed with excellent angiographic response (**Fig. 2**). Over the next few months, the blood pressure regimen was titrated down to 2 medicines, and is presently well controlled (resting blood pressure, 119/80 mm Hg) on 2 mg of perindopril and 2.5 mg of bisoprolol, 3 years after the angioplasty. She continues to have residual left hemiparesis, and serial imaging revealed complete obliteration of the right MCA with encephalomalacia in the corresponding perfused territory.

SCREENING FOR FIBROMUSCULAR RENAL ARTERY STENOSIS: FOR WHOM, WHEN, AND WHY?

Before answering this question, it is important to address the prevalence and the natural history (clinical manifestation) of FMD.

Population Prevalence

Renovascular hypertension is thought to be the cause of hypertension in about 1% to 2% of patients with hypertension. Among these, most (about 80%–90%) cases are caused by atherosclerotic renal artery stenosis, leaving perhaps 10% to 20% with renal FMD. Assuming a population prevalence of hypertension of 20%, this would lead to a crude estimate of renal FMD in the population of about 0.4%.[6] However, data from the literature suggest otherwise. The prevalence of FMD among potential kidney donors who underwent either a conventional or CT renal angiogram is reported to be between 2% and 6.6%.[8–10] The renal transplant donor population is different from the general population, and extrapolation of these numbers may represent an underestimate (because donors are usually screened out for hypertension and kidney disease) or an overestimate (because they are more likely family members of someone with severe kidney disease). For the Cardiovascular Outcomes in Renal Atherosclerotic Lesions (CORAL) trial, which included patients with atherosclerotic renal artery stenosis, 87 of the 4375 subjects initially screened were excluded for having FMD.[11] Of the 997 subjects who underwent renal angiogram, 58 (5.8%) were noted to have hitherto undiagnosed FMD, with a marked gender difference (8.6% among women, 2.8% among men).[11] However, this population was also different from the general population, being older individuals with hypertension. An autopsy series of 819 consecutive autopsies from the Mayo Clinic reported 9 cases of renal FMD (corresponding with 1.1% prevalence).[12] Despite the exact prevalence of FMD in the general population not being known, these studies suggest that it is frequently asymptomatic, or with vague symptoms that are disregarded, and hence undetected, and that it is a less rare entity than was previously thought.

Of course, compared with the general population, the prevalence is higher in hypertensive patients. Additional patient characteristics might help to further narrow the patient population at higher risk of FMD. In contrast with earlier dogmas that this disease is more prevalent among young women of Asian origin, it is unclear whether it varies by ethnic or racial groups. However, data

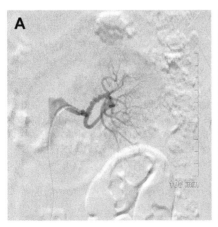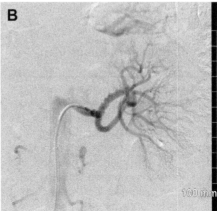

Fig. 1. (*A*) Selective left renal angiography, showing beaded appearance with multiple webs consistent with fibromuscular dysplasia within the terminal left renal artery and continuing throughout the length of a large upper pole branch. (*B*) Left renal artery angiographic images after angioplasty of the left upper pole branch.

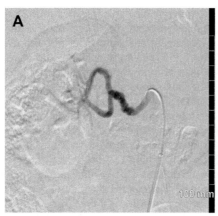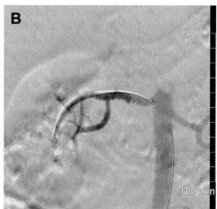

Fig. 2. (*A*) Right renal angiography showing beaded appearance involving distal two-thirds of the main renal artery and extending for a short distance into the large first-order branch to the upper pole. (*B*) Right renal angiographic images after angioplasty of the main renal artery and upper pole branch.

from the US registry and the French data support the female preponderance, by a ratio of about 9:1 (possibly related to higher progesterone expression in renovascular smooth muscle cells).[13] Although classically described as a disease that affects women of childbearing age, the average 4-year delay from the initial diagnosis of hypertension results in an average age of FMD diagnosis in the early 50s.[7,14] FMD has also rarely been reported in infancy and in the very elderly.[7,15] A family history of FMD is common, with self-reported (hence possibly an underestimate) data for first-degree or second-degree relatives in 7% to 11%,[10,16] although a much higher rate of 60% was reported in a smaller study with a formal pedigree analysis.[17] In addition, family history may be significant for other reasons: sudden death (20%), stroke (53.5%), and vascular aneurysm (23.5%) are more common in families of patients with diagnosed FMD.[14] Whether these familial events reflect missed FMD diagnoses or some other common pathogenic mechanism is not known presently.

Common Presentations of Fibromuscular Dysplasia

Although hypertension is the most common clinical presentation, the presence of headache (reported in about half) and pulsatile tinnitus (a quarter) is common. Other symptoms that are seen less commonly include flank or abdominal pain and depend on the vascular bed that is involved. Some of these symptoms, such as pulsatile tinnitus, may be accompanied by headache and neck pain but in the absence of hypertension, making the diagnosis of FMD treacherous for unwary clinicians. Fatigue and unspecified myalgia are also common symptoms, perhaps supported

by data suggesting there is more widespread connective tissue involvement.[18] Physical examination can provide additional clues, chiefly the presence of vascular bruits, which have a high specificity.[14]

Aneurysms (about 1 in 5) and dissections (about 1 in 4) in the vascular bed are often seen, with carotid and intracranial bed being the most commonly affected, followed by renal arteries and the aorta.[19] Again, this might not be an accurate estimate, because imaging often is performed more frequently in symptomatic patients. Most vascular beds have been reported to be involved, including coronary, vertebral, iliopopliteal, and subclavian arteries. Depending on the location, the clinical manifestation can range from being severe, including stroke, such as the case described earlier (FMD is responsible for about 20% of strokes in patents aged <45 years) or may even be completely asymptomatic.[19] Paradoxically, registry data suggest that the presence of vascular dissection results in a diagnosis of FMD at an earlier age (lead time of about 5 years compared with those with renal FMD alone), probably stemming from a search caused by the presentation of an acute dissection. In addition, spontaneous coronary artery dissection (SCAD) has been strongly associated with FMD.[14] Although overall it is rare, with a reported incidence of 0.2% to 1.1% in angiographic series, SCAD could be present in up to 25% of young women presenting with acute coronary syndrome.[20]

From Pathologic to Angiographic Classification

With respect to the classification, the histologic version (most common type being medial FMD with its distinctive subtypes of medial fibroplasia, perimedial fibroplasia, and medial hyperplasia, followed by intimal fibroplasia and adventitial disease) has been taken over by the angiographic version (**Table 1**). Because this disease is now almost exclusively diagnosed radiographically, and open surgery with access to renal arterial tissue is rare, use of the older histopathologic classification is limited. The angiographic classification, now endorsed by European Consensus and by the American Heart Association, classifies FMD as focal or multifocal.[21,22] Multifocal disease is the classic string-of-beads appearance represented by medial fibroplasia in virtually all adults, and is much more common (~80% of all cases of FMD).[21] Focal disease (irrespective of the length of the lesion) is usually caused by intimal hyperplasia (and less likely by medial hyperplasia and adventitial FMD). Other clinical characteristics also are different, with younger age at developing hypertension and diagnosis for focal disease, and more likelihood of having bilateral renal as well as extrarenal involvement in multifocal disease.[21]

Age and Screening: What Should Be the Thresholds?

The intersection of the increasing incidence of both obesity and essential hypertension with the commonly reported age at diagnosis for FMD creates a dilemma, making screening decisions difficult based on age alone. The overall prevalence of hypertension in the general population is slowly increasing, from 28.9% in 2009 to 33.5% in 2014. The prevalence of hypertension in adolescence (ages 8–17 years) is also increasing compared with 1988 to 2008; 15.8% to 19.2% in boys and 8.2% to 12.6% in girls.[23] Increasing obesity (body mass index and waist circumference) and salt intake were significant explanatory variables for this increase. In childhood, obesity also increases with age, with a doubling of obesity from ages 2 to 5 years (12% in boys and 8% in girls) to ages 12 to 19 years (20% in boys and 19% in girls).[24] The convergence of these lifestyle factors and obesity with hypertension means that most young individuals with newly diagnosed hypertension still do not have FMD. However, the data from the donor studies discussed earlier (2%–6.6% prevalence of FMD) as well as from the CORAL trial (5.8% in those eligible who underwent a renal angiogram) show the possible extent of the underdiagnosis of FMD. Moreover, Trinquart and colleagues[25] showed that the younger the patient, and the shorter the duration of hypertension, the greater the likelihood of cure of hypertension in FMD with angioplasty or surgical bypass. A delayed diagnosis may lead to resistant or even refractory hypertension. In addition, the opportunity for a cure may be lost, with the lifelong burden of taking antihypertensive medications. Hence testing for renal FMD in newly diagnosed hypertensive individuals has material consequences for management and treatment outcomes. Hence, screening for asymptomatic patients, especially women, more than 20 years of age who have been newly diagnosed with hypertension is a reasonable strategy. There needs to be a ceiling, however, because the prevalence of essential hypertension increases with increasing age. Hence, it is prudent to not screen asymptomatic individuals with newly diagnosed essential hypertension beyond a certain age, perhaps 50 years, given the average age of hypertension onset in patients with diagnosed FMD. Importantly, the presence of any other concerning symptoms, signs, and the presence of family history (of FMD, or sudden death and stroke) should warrant screening even outside this age range, as explained later. With increasing age, especially

Table 1
Classification of fibromuscular dysplasia: from pathology to angiography

	Focal	Multifocal
Pathologic classification	Commonly intimal fibroplasia	Commonly medial fibroplasia
Angiographic appearance	Presence of a single focal or tubular stenosis	Presence of ≥2 stenoses on a given vessel segment with or without the typical string-of-beads appearance
Clinical presentation	Usually younger age at presentation, with higher blood pressure Renal asymmetry more common; more likely to have intervention	More commonly affects multiple vascular trees, including bilateral renal lesions

Data from Savard S, Steichen O, Azarine A, et al. Association between 2 angiographic subtypes of renal artery fibromuscular dysplasia and clinical characteristics. Circulation 2012;126(25):3062–9.

beyond 50 years, and more so beyond 60 years, the likelihood of patients with asymptomatic newly diagnosed hypertension having FMD decreases exponentially. However, clinicians should take into account aneurysms and dissections as part of the natural history of FMD, and also that in, two-thirds of patients, the disease involves more than 1 artery. That realization directly leads to a second question: why should clinicians screen for FMD of renal arteries? The evidence indicating that awareness of FMD in renal vascular bed could prevent adverse vascular outcomes of otherwise undiagnosed renal lesions as well as undiagnosed and asymptomatic extrarenal lesions is discussed later.

WHEN A MISSED DIAGNOSIS SPELLS CATASTROPHE: EXTRARENAL FIBROMUSCULAR DYSPLASIA
Cerebrovascular Fibromuscular Dysplasia

Findings from the US Registry for Fibromuscular Dysplasia suggest that extrarenal FMD is nearly as prevalent as disease involving renal arteries (discussed earlier).[14] Symptoms and signs of the disease in the extrarenal arterial bed may be even less specific than those associated with FMD of renal arteries. To complicate matters further, adverse vascular outcomes of a missed diagnosis of extrarenal FMD are much more catastrophic, as seen in the case discussed earlier. In the US registry, headache (52%), pulsatile tinnitus (27%), neck pain (22%), and dizziness (26%) were the reported symptoms of the cerebrovascular (carotid and vertebral arteries) disease.[14] Cervical bruit (22%) was the most common presenting diagnostic sign. Reported association between carotid artery FMD and aneurysm formation is 21% and is lower for FMD in other cerebrovascular territories, such as cerebral (11%), basilar (7%), and vertebral (3%).[14] The association between cerebrovascular FMD and dissection is even stronger than for disease involving renal arteries: 75% for carotid artery and 17% for vertebral artery.[14,19] Overall, the prevalence of cerebrovascular aneurysms in the US registry was 7%. From a different perspective, up to 15% to 20% of patients with reported spontaneous dissection of the carotid vertebral arteries have FMD.[20] Clinical sequelae of cerebrovascular FMD include transient ischemic attack and stroke, amaurosis fugax, subarachnoid hemorrhage, and focal neurologic symptoms caused by stenosis-related hypoperfusion/ischemia, embolization, thrombosis, dissection, and aneurysm rupture. These conditions can have serious long-term sequelae, given that they occur in young patients with otherwise productive lives ahead of them, as seen in the case report earlier.

Fibromuscular Dysplasia in Other Vascular Beds

With regard to extrarenal and extracerebrovascular FMD, mesenteric ischemia is an uncommon manifestation of FMD, seen in only 1.8% of patients.[14,19] Mesenteric/celiac disease accounted for 6.8% of all arterial dissections and 22.3% of aneurysms in this registry. FMD of coronary arteries is rarely diagnosed as the typical appearance of the string of beads. Instead, distal tapering, focal stenosis, tortuosity, and dissection of otherwise nonatherosclerotic coronary arteries may raise suspicion of FMD. Acute coronary syndrome secondary to FMD seems to be rare from the small numbers of cases ever reported; however, the report of a strong association of SCAD with FMD should be considered in young women who present with an acute coronary syndrome.[20] In addition, claudication and acute ischemia of lower and upper extremities have been reported secondary to aneurysms, dissection, and thromboembolic events associated with iliac, subclavian, and brachial FMD.

Overall, the catastrophic consequences of a missed diagnosis of extrarenal FMD, especially when involving the cerebrovascular territory, should prompt physicians for early diagnosis and intervention in patients with symptoms, signs, or significant family history.

Renal and Extrarenal Fibromuscular Dysplasia: Which Imaging Tests and When?

Screening for FMD is primarily with imaging tests; namely Doppler ultrasonography, CT angiography, and magnetic resonance (MR) angiography. The confirmatory gold standard for diagnosis is conventional or catheter angiography. However, there are no population-wide screening data, such as for screening of newly diagnosed hypertensive patients (asymptomatic or otherwise), at different age groups with these 3 modalities, or confirmation with angiography, to provide accurate positive and negative predictive values or likelihood ratios. The authors suggest considering the potential risk, cost, and local expertise along with the diagnostic yield when choosing the imaging test for screening.[26]

Doppler Ultrasonography

Renal FMD mostly involves the mid and distal parts of the renal artery and may also involve branches of main renal artery. Doppler ultrasonography, in highly skilled hands, showing step-up in peak systolic velocity in the mid to distal portion of the renal artery or a delayed systolic upstroke in the main artery or its branches distal to the stenosis, is highly accurate.[27] However, it loses its sensitivity for the terminal portion of the main renal artery and its branches. It is also time consuming and highly operator dependent, making its use in clinical practice further limited.[27,28] However, follow-up of renal FMD postintervention can easily be performed with Doppler ultrasonography.

Computed Tomography Angiography

CT angiography is fast, and less operator dependent, but it involves radiation and contrast exposure. A single acquisition can easily include the neck, chest, abdomen, and peripheral vessels. Additional advantages of CT angiography include the visualization of the vessel wall and renal parenchyma in addition to the vessel lumen.[26] Although an older study suggests moderate sensitivity (64% compared with conventional angiography),[29] progress in technology in the last decade suggests that CT angiography can be considered acceptable for screening.

Magnetic Resonance Angiography

MR angiography does not need radiation, nor does it require iodinated contrast, and the use of gadolinium, if necessary, should be mostly possible given the preserved kidney function in most patients with FMD. MR angiography can also delineate vessel wall and renal parenchyma, and although its spatial resolution renders distal renal artery visualization limited, newer techniques can overcome these limitations.[30] Subtle motion artifacts, longer time (compared with CT angiography acquisition), and higher cost are additional limitations.[26]

Consideration of Extrarenal Fibromuscular Dysplasia

For extrarenal FMD screening and diagnosis, both CT and MR angiography are advantageous in offering faster acquisition compared with Doppler. Another limitation of the Doppler is access to extrarenal sites that may have disease, such as the intracranial stretch of the carotid circulation. Dissections and aneurysms can be potentially diagnosed by all 3 modalities, with the caveats of MR angiography being less accurate for smaller aneurysms (<6 mm), and Doppler being operator dependent. There are insufficient data on the sensitivity and specificity of these imaging modalities for extrarenal FMD diagnosis at present.

Screening Approach

- Thus, a renal-limited Doppler may be sufficient for screening if easily available when screening in asymptomatic young women with newly diagnosed hypertension, with CT or MR angiography as an acceptable follow-up confirmatory test. In cases in which the index of suspicion is higher and intervention is being considered, renal Doppler could be followed directly by conventional angiography and angioplasty.
- In the presence of suspicious symptoms (eg, pulsatile tinnitus) or signs (eg, neck or flank bruits), when the likelihood of FMD is higher, more extensive CT or MR angiography should be considered as the superior initial screening test. These tests also allow better diagnosis of FMD at extrarenal sites.
- Most importantly, because extrarenal FMD is more common than was previously thought, the diagnosis of renal FMD should prompt an initial screen with CT or MR angiography for extrarenal FMD in all patients. In addition, there should be a low threshold for repeat imaging with the development of new symptoms or signs in patients with initial renal-limited FMD.

REFERENCES

1. Goldblatt H, Lynch J, Hanzal RF, et al. Studies on experimental hypertension: I. The production of persistent elevation of systolic blood pressure by means of renal ischemia. J Exp Med 1934;59(3): 347–79.
2. Leadbetter WF, Dodson, Burkland C. Hypertension in unilateral renal disease. J Urol 1938;39(5):611–26.
3. Meaney TF, Dodson AE, Poutasse EF, et al. Observations concerning renal circulation: angiography of kidneys, removed from hypertensive or normotensive patients. Cleve Clin Q 1958;25(1):21–31.
4. Harrison EG Jr, McCormack LJ. Pathologic classification of renal arterial disease in renovascular hypertension. Mayo Clin Proc 1971;46(3):161–7.
5. Weinberg I, Gu X, Giri J, et al. Anti-platelet and anti-hypertension medication use in patients with fibromuscular dysplasia: results from the United States Registry for Fibromuscular Dysplasia. Vasc Med 2015;20(5):447–53.
6. Plouin PF, Perdu J, La Batide-Alanore A, et al. Fibromuscular dysplasia. Orphanet J Rare Dis 2007;2:28.
7. Olin JW, Gornik HL, Bacharach JM, et al. Fibromuscular dysplasia: state of the science and critical unanswered questions: a scientific statement from the American Heart Association. Circulation 2014; 129(9):1048–78.

8. Frick MP, Goldberg ME. Uro- and angiographic findings in a "normal" population: screening of 151 symptom-free potential transplant donors for renal disease. AJR Am J Roentgenol 1980;134(3):503–5.

9. Neymark E, LaBerge JM, Hirose R, et al. Arteriographic detection of renovascular disease in potential renal donors: incidence and effect on donor surgery. Radiology 2000;214(3):755–60.

10. Shivapour DM, Erwin P, Kim E. Epidemiology of fibromuscular dysplasia: a review of the literature. Vasc Med 2016;21(4):376–81.

11. Cooper CJ, Murphy TP, Cutlip DE, et al. Stenting and medical therapy for atherosclerotic renal-artery stenosis. N Engl J Med 2014;370(1):13–22.

12. Heffelfinger M, Holley KE, Harrison EG Jr, et al. Arterial fibromuscular dysplasia studied at autopsy. Am J Clin Pathol 1970;54:274.

13. Silhol F, Sarlon-Bartoli G, Daniel L, et al. Intranuclear expression of progesterone receptors in smooth muscle cells of renovascular fibromuscular dysplasia: a pilot study. Ann Vasc Surg 2015;29(4):830–5.

14. Olin JW, Froehlich J, Gu X, et al. The United States Registry for Fibromuscular Dysplasia: results in the first 447 patients. Circulation 2012;125(25):3182–90.

15. Green R, Gu X, Kline-Rogers E, et al. Differences between the pediatric and adult presentation of fibromuscular dysplasia: results from the US registry. Pediatr Nephrol 2016;31(4):641–50.

16. Pannier-Moreau I, Grimbert P, Fiquet-Kempf B, et al. Possible familial origin of multifocal renal artery fibromuscular dysplasia. J Hypertens 1997;15(12 Pt 2):1797–801.

17. Rushton AR. The genetics of fibromuscular dysplasia. Arch Intern Med 1980;140(2):233–6.

18. Ganesh SK, Morissette R, Xu Z, et al. Clinical and biochemical profiles suggest fibromuscular dysplasia is a systemic disease with altered TGF-beta expression and connective tissue features. FASEB J 2014;28(8):3313–24.

19. Kadian-Dodov D, Gornik HL, Gu X, et al. Dissection and aneurysm in patients with fibromuscular dysplasia: findings from the U.S. registry for FMD. J Am Coll Cardiol 2016;68(2):176–85.

20. Saw J, Aymong E, Mancini GB, et al. Nonatherosclerotic coronary artery disease in young women. Can J Cardiol 2014;30(7):814–9.

21. Savard S, Steichen O, Azarine A, et al. Association between 2 angiographic subtypes of renal artery fibromuscular dysplasia and clinical characteristics. Circulation 2012;126(25):3062–9.

22. Persu A, Touze E, Mousseaux E, et al. Diagnosis and management of fibromuscular dysplasia: an expert consensus. Eur J Clin Invest 2012;42(3):338–47.

23. Rosner B, Cook NR, Daniels S, et al. Childhood blood pressure trends and risk factors for high blood pressure: the NHANES experience 1988-2008. Hypertension 2013;62(2):247–54.

24. Ogden CL, Carroll MD, Kit BK, et al. Prevalence of childhood and adult obesity in the United States, 2011-2012. JAMA 2014;311(8):806–14.

25. Trinquart L, Mounier-Vehier C, Sapoval M, et al. Efficacy of revascularization for renal artery stenosis caused by fibromuscular dysplasia: a systematic review and meta-analysis. Hypertension 2010;56(3):525–32.

26. Lewis S, Kadian-Dodov D, Bansal A, et al. Multimodality imaging of fibromuscular dysplasia. Abdom Radiol (NY) 2016;41(10):2048–60.

27. Olin JW, Piedmonte MR, Young JR, et al. The utility of duplex ultrasound scanning of the renal arteries for diagnosing significant renal artery stenosis. Ann Intern Med 1995;122(11):833–8.

28. Riehl J, Schmitt H, Bongartz D, et al. Renal artery stenosis: evaluation with colour duplex ultrasonography. Nephrol Dial Transplant 1997;12(8):1608–14.

29. Vasbinder GB, Nelemans PJ, Kessels AG, et al. Accuracy of computed tomographic angiography and magnetic resonance angiography for diagnosing renal artery stenosis. Ann Intern Med 2004;141(9):674–82 [discussion: 682].

30. Glockner JF, Takahashi N, Kawashima A, et al. Noncontrast renal artery MRA using an inflow inversion recovery steady state free precession technique (Inhance): comparison with 3D contrast-enhanced MRA. J Magn Reson Imaging 2010;31(6):1411–8.

Device-Directed Therapy for Resistant Hypertension

Sinan S. Tankut, MD*, Ayhan Yoruk, MD, MPH,
John D. Bisognano, MD, PhD

KEYWORDS

- Resistant hypertension • Renal denervation • Baroreceptor activation therapy
- Median nerve stimulation

KEY POINTS

- Hypertension is a chronic medical condition with increasing risk for renal, cerebrovascular, and cardiovascular disease if left untreated.
- Of patients with diagnosis of hypertension, 20% to 30% have uncontrolled blood pressures despite appropriate medical management.
- Innovative techniques such as renal denervation therapy, baroreceptor activation therapy, and median nerve stimulation therapies are potential solutions for the management of resistant hypertension.

Hypertension, the most prevalent chronic disease worldwide, is a major risk factor for vision loss, renal disease, cardiovascular and cerebrovascular illnesses. Approximately 70 million Americans, that is one out of every three adults, are diagnosed with hypertension. With only about half of this population having their condition under control, the economic burden was projected to be $46 billion in 2011.[1] With such a significant impact on society, there have been tremendous efforts and continued progress toward tackling this issue in the last century. Historically, surgical approaches such as sympathectomies and nerve stimulation[2,3] have provided encouraging results for lowering blood pressure. However, due to the high incidence of procedural and long-term complications, as well as the irreversible nature of such surgical operations, the focus on managing hypertension has since transitioned to pharmacologic agents, including sympatholytic agents, calcium channel blockers, diuretics, and ACE inhibitors/angiotensin receptor blockers.

Despite the availability of various drug classes, a large number of patients fail to achieve goal blood pressures. Resistant hypertension is defined as blood pressure that is persistently above goal (<140/90 mmHg for most patients) despite the use of maximally tolerated doses of three different antihypertensive medications, one being a diuretic. The prevalence of resistant hypertension is estimated to be approximately 20% to 30% among the population with a known diagnosis of hypertension.[4] With the aging population, increasing rates of obesity, and sedentary lifestyle, the incidence of resistant hypertension is expected to increase. There are several reasons why individuals develop resistant hypertension. First, patients can falsely be categorized with resistant hypertension secondary to issues with medication adherence in the setting of

Disclosure Statement: J.D. Bisognano received consultant and research support from CVRx.
University of Rochester Medical Center, 601 Elmwood Avenue, PO Box MED, Rochester, NY 14642, USA
* Corresponding author.
E-mail address: Sinan_Tankut@urmc.rochester.edu

cardiology.theclinics.com

polypharmacy and barriers to accessing health care. Per Tomaszewski and colleagues,[5] up to 25% to 65% of the population is nonadherent to their antihypertensive therapy. Second, despite the appropriate management of hypertension, patients remain on medications such as nonsteroidal antiinflammatory drugs, amphetamines, and nasal decongestants that are known to contribute to elevated blood pressures. Additionally, chronic medical conditions such as heart failure and kidney disease may present with persistently elevated blood pressures unless these conditions are properly managed. Finally, chronic pain and stress, along with undiagnosed secondary hypertension from conditions such as obstructive sleep apnea, renal artery stenosis, pheochromocytoma, hypothyroidism or hyperthyroidism, and many more could potentially interfere with proper hypertension management while on maximum pharmacotherapy.[6] There is strong evidence to suggest that lowering blood pressure can reduce the risk of certain illnesses such as cardiovascular disease or stroke.[7] Therefore, the role of device-directed interventions such as renal denervation therapy, baroreceptor activation therapy (BAT), and median nerve stimulators are crucial and, perhaps in certain cases, necessary in the setting of resistant hypertension. There are ongoing research efforts to improve these innovative devices, with a keen focus on therapeutic efficacy and safety to best manage resistant hypertension. The following is a review of these innovative interventions.

RENAL DENERVATION

The kidneys have several mechanisms to regulate blood pressure, with several pharmaceutical options available to influence this regulation. Medications such as ACE inhibitors/angiotensin receptor blockers that disrupt the angiotensin-renin pathway and diuretics that prevent water reabsorption are already used extensively. However, evidence demonstrating an interplay between renal sympathetic activity and hypertension has brought about device-directed therapies for blood pressure control, including renal denervation therapy. This treatment modality consists consists of advancing a catheter to the renal arteries, which are in close proximity to the renal nerves. Energy, mostly in the form of radiofrequency, is released from the catheter with goals to achieve denervation, thus inhibiting the sympathetic pathway and lowering blood pressure.[8,9]

This promising approach to disrupting sympathetic input through the renal nerves led to the Symplicity Hypertension (HTN) trials. Symplicity HTN-1 was a prospective, single-arm study that monitored blood pressure readings for 45 subjects who had met the criteria for resistant hypertension and undergone renal denervation. The study aimed to monitor in-office blood pressure readings at incremental months up to a year following the procedure. The significant outcome from the study was the immediate reduction of in-office blood pressure readings (systolic blood pressure [SBP] −14 and diastolic blood pressure [DBP] −10 mmHg) after the first month and its sustained effect after 12 months (SBP −27 and DBP −17 mmHg). These were encouraging results and heralded advancing therapies for resistant hypertension. However, due to the small sample size and statistically insignificant reduction of ambulatory blood pressure in a relatively small subset (n = 9, SBP −11 mmHg), more research on a larger sample size was necessary to validate the success of renal denervation.[8–10]

The subsequent study, the Symplicity HTN-2 trial, included a larger sample size of 106 subjects who again met the criteria for resistant hypertension. Additionally, this trial was the first randomized trial to compare the therapeutic benefits of renal denervation (52 subjects) versus standard antihypertensive medications (54 subjects). The Symplicity HTN-2 trial demonstrated superior therapeutic outcomes at the six month in-office blood pressure readings for the group that underwent renal denervation therapy (SBP −32 and DBP −12 mmHg) compared with the group that was on traditional antihypertensive medications (SBP −0 and DBP −1 mmHg). Despite these promising results, including improvement of in-office blood pressure readings, as well as minimizing adverse events from the procedures, these two trials failed to show improvement of 24-hour ambulatory blood pressure.[9–11] The EnligHTN-1 was another trial that evaluated the efficacy and safety of renal denervation therapy delivered via advanced multi-electrode system. The study consisted of 46 subjects with resistant hypertension with goals to monitor in-office blood pressure readings up to 6 months after implementation. The trial demonstrated good results with immediate (1-month SBP −28 and DBP −10 mmHg) and sustained (6-month SBP −26 and DBP −10 mmHg) in-office blood pressure reductions. However, similar to the Symplicity HTN trials, EnligHTN-1 failed to show any significant changes in 24-hour ambulatory blood pressure readings (6-months SBP −10 and DBP −6 mmHg).[12] The cause remains unclear for the difference between in-office and 24-hour ambulatory blood pressure readings. In an extensive review conducted by investigators Li and colleagues,[9] factors including the white coat effect, medication adherence, and inclusion of subjects with undiagnosed secondary hypertension could have potentially played a role in the significant difference between the groups. Further research is warranted to further explore the differences in these findings. Additionally, future research should focus on more reliable outcomes.

The Symplicity HTN-3 trial was designed to evaluate renal denervation therapy in conjunction with optimal medication therapy in a larger population with resistant hypertension against a placebo group that underwent sham procedure. The outcomes were disappointing because there was no difference in 24-hour ambulatory or in-office blood pressure readings between the two groups.[13]

The Symplicity HTN-4 trial is currently underway with enrollment of subjects in 2014. This particular study aims to follow-up on the failure of the previous trial by modifying the inclusion criteria and investigating the optimal degree of ablation needed to reach denervation. Symplicity HTN-3 was exclusively aimed at subjects with uncontrolled hypertension with SBP greater than 160 mmHg despite pharmacotherapy. This criterion will be relaxed to include subjects with SBP ranging from 140 to 160 mmHg. Again, a question raised following the Symplicity HTN-3 trial was the degree of ablation needed to achieve denervation. To prevent postoperative complications such as renal artery stenosis, a conservative amount of radiofrequency was delivered to the renal nerves. Therefore, the amount of radiofrequency delivered to reach therapeutic denervation from previous trials has been questioned. One of the aims for Symplicity HTN-4 will be to determine the optimal degree of ablation necessary for renal nerve denervation to have a therapeutic outcome and maintain its established safety profile.[14]

BARORECEPTOR ACTIVATION THERAPY

Baroreceptors are integral components in the regulation of the body's hemodynamics. Physiologically, baroreceptors in the carotid sinus and aortic arch sense mechanical stretching of the arterial walls, which in turn leads to changes in the sympathetic nervous system, a large component of circulatory physiology. Inhibiting sympathetic signaling leads to an increase in parasympathetic activity, with subsequent lowering of blood pressure. Innovate therapies aiming to harness this ability to modulate the sympathetic system, through the stimulation of baroreceptors, have been evaluated through clinical trials.

The Device-Based Therapy in Hypertension Trial (DEBuT-HT) was the first single-arm human trial that tested the safety and efficacy of implantable iatrogenic BAT on human subjects. The initial device consisted of two pulse generators that were surgically implanted around the carotid bulbs bilaterally along with a pulse generator in the pectoralis region. The study consisted of 45 individuals with a diagnosis of resistant hypertension. The results were promising, demonstrating reduction of blood pressure at three months (SBP −21 and DBP −12 mmHg), one year (SBP −30 and −20 mmHg), and two years (SBP −33 and DBP −22 mmHg).[15]

Following these encouraging results from the DEBuT-HT, there was a need to further evaluate device therapy within a larger population against a placebo group. The Rheos Pivotal Trial involved 265 subjects and was the first randomized, double-blinded study conducted to further evaluate BAT. All subjects had CVRx Rheos device implantation and were randomized into two separate groups. Subjects who visited their physician's office after one month would either have their device turned on at that time or alternatively would have their device turned on after a six month follow-up. Timing of device activation was five months off between two groups in an effort to evaluate the acute efficacy of BAT. Despite the encouraging findings from the DEBuT-HT, the trial failed to show statistical difference in blood pressure reduction at six months, bringing into question the therapy's acute efficacy. Additionally, the trial failed to meet the predetermined procedural safety criteria, raising further concerns for the use of BAT. However, the study did demonstrate sustained blood pressure reduction in those who responded to therapy with an average 25 mmHg SBP reduction in both groups.[16,17] Given these results, the trial was extended for long-term monitoring of the 271 subjects who successfully responded to CVRx Rheos device implantation. During the average follow-up of 28 months, with a maximum of 53 months, the reduction in blood pressure that was demonstrated at 12 months was maintained throughout.[18] Furthermore, these subjects also demonstrated a reduction in the number of antihypertensive medications used.

The Barostim neo (CVRx) is an improved second-generation device aiming to improve on the original Rheos device, consisting of a smaller pulse generator with a single electrode that is implanted unilaterally, therefore reducing the risk for procedural-related adverse events. The Barostim neo trial was the first study to evaluate BAT via unilateral stimulation of the carotid sinus for blood pressure management. The study population was fairly small, consisting of only 30 subjects with the diagnosis of resistant hypertension. The study results demonstrated a reduction in blood pressure at three months (SBP −26.1 mmHg) as well as six months (SBP −26 mmHg).[17,19] A follow-up study conducted by Wallbach and colleagues[20] monitored ambulatory blood pressure measurements in 51 subjects who were treated with the Barostim neo device. This study demonstrated statistically significant reduction of ambulatory blood pressure with 55% of the subjects having a reduction of SBP greater than or equal to 5 mmHg after six months.

Studies to date have shown promising results with BAT. The evolvement of unilateral carotid artery stimulation reduces surgical site exposure and perioperative risk. However, further research in a larger population is necessary to solidify results from previous studies. The Barostim neo Hypertension Pivotal Trial is a prospective, randomized, controlled, multicenter trial currently taking place involving approximately 310 subjects. The study will test the safety and efficacy of Barostim neo in combination with optimal medical management for resistant hypertension through a three-year follow-up of subjects.[21]

MEDIAN NERVE MODULATORS

Research efforts continue to pursue the development of and optimization of innovative therapies for resistant hypertension, with a focus on therapeutic benefit (acute vs chronic), procedural safety, and the minimization of long-term device-related complications. A relatively newer device, the Electroceutical Coin (eCoin) (Valencia Technologies, California), is a minimally invasive device aimed to treat resistant hypertension. Studies have shown that electroacupuncture via stimulation to peripheral nerves leads to a reduction in blood pressure.[22] Several studies have also illustrated that stimulation of the median nerve can result in lowering of blood pressure through modulation of the sympathetic nervous system.[23]

The median nerves are modulated via two coin-sized stimulators that are implemented subcutaneously close to the median nerve. The device produces intermittent, low-frequency stimulation to the median nerve resulting in a sympathetic inhibitory effect, which leads to vasodilation and subsequent lowering of blood pressure.[24]

A randomized, prospective, double-blinded, sham-controlled study on 48 individuals has been completed with an abstract available to detail preliminary results.[25] Two groups were divided evenly: group A subjects had their device activated after their one month follow-up and group B, the placebo group, had their device activated after six months. The six month postactivation results for all 41 subjects who were able to follow through with the study showed an in-office blood pressure reduction of −10.31 plus or minus 20.93 mmHg and a minimal decrease in 24-hour ambulatory readings (SBP −4.68 ± 11.05 mmHg). Historically, many studies have demonstrated the effectiveness of electroacupuncture on peripheral nerves for blood pressure control. However, this is among the first studies of an implantable device conducted on human subjects that evaluates median nerve modulation as a therapy for resistant hypertension.

DISCUSSION AND FUTURE TRENDS

Resistant hypertension is an ongoing threat to our society, particularly as the prevalence continues to rise. The trend toward continued research and development of novel nonpharmacological agents to tackle this issue is encouraging. Renal denervation therapy is among the most studied treatments aimed for resistant hypertension management. Initial studies such as the Symplicity HTN-1 and Symplicity HTN-2 were promising; however, Symplicity HTN-3 failed to provide concrete evidence of therapeutic benefit of renal denervation for the management of resistant hypertension. The Symplicity HTN-4 trial aims to evaluate renal denervation therapy in a slightly different population (SBP ranging between 140 and 160 mmHg) and to adjust the amount of ablation needed to achieve denervation.

The Barostim neo Hypertension Pivotal Trial aims to address issues brought up from previous clinical trials that studied the efficacy and safety of BAT. Median nerve modulation was initially described in eastern traditional medicine such as electroacupuncture and in experimental studies. However, the utility of this pioneering device therapy at this time warrants further discussion.

To date, research has mostly been conducted on devices as sole therapy for the management of resistant hypertension. A recent study conducted in Germany examined 28 subjects who received BAT following inadequate blood pressure control via renal denervation therapy. The single-arm study showed that most of the subjects reached goals of lowering in-office SBP more than 10 mmHg at 6 months (68%) and maintained these findings a year after the procedure (77%). Again the discrepancy between in-office and ambulatory blood pressure goals was evident because only 48% of the subjects reached reduction of ambulatory SBP by 5 mmHg or more at six months. Even though this study consists of a small population size, it outlined the possibility of strategies for combination device therapy. Furthermore, the discrepancy of in-office blood pressure findings and 24-hour ambulatory results outlined by previous studies warrants further analysis.[26] Additionally, the authors believe further research needs to focus on the combination of traditional therapies with these advanced devices, used as an essential adjunct to tackle this costly and devastating disease. Finally, the long-term safety profile and sustained efficacy (10-plus years) of these devices needs to be evaluated once immediate therapeutic benefit is achieved.

Hypertension is indeed a silent killer, with which patients with poorly controlled blood pressures remain at increased risk for poor health outcomes. Pharmacotherapy and lifestyle modifications remain the primary tools for blood pressure control and management. The increasing awareness of resistant hypertension and device-directed therapy creates optimism for both patients and providers in regard to the management of resistant hypertension. Continued advancements in implantable devices for the treatment of hypertension are promising, though they remain controversial due to their cost and overall effectiveness. In the progressively dynamic health care arena, continued advancements of these therapies and their ability to effectively manage resistant hypertension can be expected. These devices are crucial for the management of resistant hypertension, and may prove beneficial for individuals facing polypharmacy, intolerance to medication side effects, or those with a history of medication noncompliance. A minimally invasive implantable device could provide a sound solution to those with medical, social, and economic barriers to the management of hypertension.

REFERENCES

1. Centers for Disease Control and Prevention. High blood pressure. Available at: https://www.cdc.gov/bloodpressure/. Accessed August 29, 2016.
2. Allen EV. Sympathectomy for essential hypertension. Circulation 1952;6:131–40.
3. Smithwick RH. Surgical treatment of hypertension. Am J Med 1949;2:81–153.
4. Calhoun DA, Jones D, Textor S, American Heart Association Professional Education Committee. Resistant hypertension: diagnosis, evaluation, and treatment. Circulation 2008;117(25):e510–26.
5. Tomaszewski M, White C, Patel P. High rates of non-adherence to antihypertensive treatment revealed by high performance liquid chromatography-tandem mass spectrometry (HP LC-MS/MS) urine analysis. Heart 2014;100(11):855–61.
6. Doroszko A, Janus A, Szahidewicz – Krupska E. Resistant hypertension. Adv Clin Exp Med 2016; 25(1):173–83.
7. Law MR, Morris JK, Wald NJ. Use of blood pressure lowering drugs in the prevention of cardiovascular disease: meta-analysis of 147 randomised trials in the context of expectations from prospective epidemiological studies. BMJ 2009;338:b1665.
8. Krum H, Schlaich M, Whitbourn R, et al. Catheter-based renal sympathetic denervation for resistant hypertension: a multicentre safety and proof-of-principle cohort study. Lancet 2009;373:1275–81.
9. Li P, Nader M, Arunagiri K, et al. Device-based therapy for drug-resistant hypertension: an update. Curr Hypertens Rep 2016;18(8):64.
10. Ng FL, Saxena M, Mahfoud F, et al. Device-based therapy for hypertension. Curr Hypertens Rep 2016;18(8):61.
11. Esler MD, Krum H, Sobotka PA, et al. Renal sympathetic denervation in patients with treatment-resistant hypertension (The Symplicity HTN- 2 Trial): a randomized controlled trial. Lancet 2010;376: 1903–9.
12. Worthley SG, Tsioufis CP, Worthley MI, et al. Safety and efficacy of a multi-electrode renal sympathetic denervation system in a resistant hypertension: the EnligHTN 1 trial. Eur Heart J 2013;34:2132–40.
13. Bhatt DL, Kandzari DE, O'Neill WW, et al. A controlled trial of renal denervation for resistant hypertension. N Engl J Med 2014;370:1393–401.
14. Renal denervation in patients with uncontrolled hypertension – SYMPLICITY HTN -4. Clinical trials.gov. Available at: https://clinicaltrials.gov/ct2/show/NCT01972139. Accessed August 29, 2016.
15. Scheffers IJ, Kroon AA, Schmidli J, et al. Novel baroreflex activation therapy in resistant hypertension: results of a European multi-center feasibility study. J Am Coll Cardiol 2010;56(15):1254–8.
16. Bisognano JD, Bakris G, Nadim MK, et al. Baroreflex activation therapy lowers blood pressure in patients with resistant hypertension: results from the double-blind, randomized, placebo-controlled rheos pivotal trial. J Am Coll Cardiol 2011;58(7):765–73.
17. Yoruk A, Bisognano JD, Gassler JP. Baroreceptor stimulation for resistant hypertension. Am J Hypertens 2016;29(12):1319–24.
18. Bakris GL, Nadim MK, Haller H, et al. Baroreflex activation therapy provides durable benefit in patients with resistant hypertension: results of long-term follow-up in the Rheos Pivotal trial. J Am Soc Hypertens 2012;6(2):152–8.
19. Hoppe UC, Brandt MC, Wachter R, et al. Minimally invasive system for baroreflex activation therapy chronically lowers blood pressure with pacemaker-like safety profile: results from the Barostim neo trial. J Am Soc Hypertens 2012;6(4):270–6.
20. Wallbach M, Lehnig LY, Schroer C, et al. Effects of baroreflex activation therapy on ambulatory blood pressure in patients with resistant hypertension. Hypertension 2016;67:701–9.
21. CVRx,Inc., CVRx Clinical Trials: US Barostim neo Hypertension Pivotal Trial Minneapolis. Available at:

http://www.cvrx.com/usa/healthcare/hypertension/clinical-trials. Accessed August 29, 2016.

22. Li P, Tjen-A-Looi SC, Cheng L, et al. Long-lasting reduction of blood pressure by electroacupunture in patients with hypertension: randomized controlled trial. Med Acupunct 2015;27(4):253–66.

23. Li P, Pitsillides KF, Rendig SV, et al. Reversal of reflex-induced myocardial ischemia by median nerve stimulation – a feline model of electroacupuncture. Circulation 1998;97:1186–94.

24. Gelfand M, Levin H. 2008 Implantable Device and Method for Treatment of Hypertension. United States Patent. Paten No US 7,373,204 B2.

25. Webster M, Valle M, Blake J, et al. Median nerve modulation: a novel approach to resistant hypertension. J Am Soc Hypertens 2016;10(4S): e6–9.

26. Wallbach M, Halbach M, Reuter H, et al. Baroreflex activation therapy in patients with prior renal denervation. J Hypertens 2016;34(8):1631–8.

Contemporary Approaches to Patients with Heart Failure

Sumeet S. Mitter, MD, MSc, Clyde W. Yancy, MD, MSc*

KEYWORDS

- Heart failure with reduced ejection fraction • Heart failure with preserved ejection fraction
- Mortality • Guideline directed medical therapy

KEY POINTS

- Cohort and Medicare data reveal that incident heart failure and hospitalization for heart failure are decreasing. Furthermore, mortality among heart failure patients is increasingly due to noncardiovascular causes.
- Current evidence-based therapy for heart failure has improved heart failure–related mortality. Current efforts should be directed toward optimizing evidence-based medical and device therapy, reducing morbidity, and increasing the number of quality life-years with heart failure.
- In addition to the use of angiotensin-converting enzyme inhibitors/angiotensin receptor blockers, beta-blockers, mineralocorticoid receptor antagonists, implantable cardiac defibrillators, and cardiac resynchronization therapy to reduce mortality for heart failure with reduced ejection fraction (HFrEF), newer evidence supports the use of angiotensin receptor–neprilysin inhibitors and sinoatrial modulators to manage chronic stage C HFrEF.
- Innovations in regenerative therapy for HFrEF remain to be seen, whereas durable mechanical support is an established standard of care for end-stage heart failure as either destination therapy or a bridge to heart transplantation.
- Heart failure with preserved ejection fraction (HFpEF) remains without a specific indicated intervention that improves the natural history. The prevailing recommendation remains a focus on the associated comorbidities, for example, hypertension, atrial fibrillation, chronic renal disease, and obesity for which evidence-based interventions have been established. Future clinical trials should focus on therapies to reduce HFpEF mortality, especially as the burden of HFpEF is expected to exceed HFrEF in the coming years.

INTRODUCTION

It is estimated that 5.7 million adults are currently living with heart failure in the United States. That number is expected to exceed 8 million by 2030 with 915,000 new cases being diagnosed annually. Annual costs for heart failure care are expected to grow from $30.7 billion to $69.7 billion by 2030 as well.[1] Moreover, 1 in 5 adults are expected to develop heart failure after the age of 40, a rate that remains constant even among adults over the age of 80 in the remaining years of their lives. It is critical then to optimize care for heart failure given the increasing prevalence and cost of heart failure.

Disclosure Statement: The authors have no relevant commercial or financial conflicts of interest.
Division of Cardiology, Department of Medicine, Northwestern University Feinberg School of Medicine, 676 North Saint Clair Street, Suite 600, Chicago, IL 60611, USA
* Corresponding author.
E-mail address: cyancy@nm.org

Although 5-year mortality after a diagnosis of heart failure exceeds 50%, noncardiovascular causes account for more than 54% of deaths in heart failure patients.[1] Further prognostication and appropriate management of any heart failure patient require an understanding that heart failure is a syndrome and not a finite illness.

Dichotomizing heart failure patients as having HFrEF, defined as heart failure and a left ventricular ejection fraction ≤40%, or HFpEF, defined as heart failure with left ventricular ejection fraction ≥50%, has vital implications for subsequent care.[2] The current understanding of heart failure syndromes is evolving, with recent data identifying a separate new entity, *heart failure with recovered ejection fraction*, with at least separate prognostic implications from HFrEF and HFpEF.[3,4]

Temporal analyses from Olmstead County in Minneapolis reveal that between 2000 and 2010, incident heart failure rates *decreased* by 4.6% annually, with a greater reduction in incident heart failure of 45% for HFrEF and 28% for HFpEF.[5] Furthermore, hospitalizations and death for individuals with heart failure were driven primarily by noncardiovascular causes with slight improvements in all-cause 30-day readmission rates among Medicare beneficiaries.[5,6] A closer look at Medicare data reveals that, nationwide, hospitalizations for heart failure are declining by 3.1% annually with an overall reduction in the rate of hospitalization for heart failure by 30.5% between 1999 and 2011.[7] In aggregate, these trends reveal an emerging shift in emphasis to heart failure with preserved ejection fraction and the growing problem of recurrent hospitalization. Mortality however is improving as evidenced by years lived with heart failure.[5]

These measured successes may be attributed to the evidence-based, contemporary approaches to the management of heart failure syndromes formalized in the 2013 joint guidelines from the American College of Cardiology Foundation (ACCF) and the American Heart Association (AHA) and in the more recently updated heart failure guidelines in the 2016 Focused Update.[2,8] Treatment of heart failure within these guidelines is recommended based on stages of heart failure, reflecting the development and progression of disease. Stage A heart failure refers to those individuals at high risk for heart failure yet exhibit no structural heart disease or symptoms of heart failure.[9] Stage B heart failure refers to those individuals with structural heart disease but who remain asymptomatic from heart failure. Stage C thus reflects those individuals with structural heart disease who were previously or are currently symptomatic. Last, stage D heart failure reflects refractory heart failure despite appropriate therapy with an increased risk for recurrent hospitalization and

death. Stage D requires specialized interventions for advanced therapy. Notably, the stages of heart failure are static categorizations and imply a unidirectional progression in disease. These stages differ from the dynamic New York Heart Association (NYHA) Functional Classification system, which relies on exercise capacity and current symptoms.[10]

Stages A and B Heart Failure

Ideally, heart failure management begins first with recognizing patients who have risk factors for heart failure, despite no apparent structural heart disease, also known as stage A heart failure. Management of stage A heart failure thus involves treating hypertension and hyperlipidemia according to contemporary guidelines in order to lower the risk for developing heart failure,[11,12] and, to a lesser degree, controlling obesity, diabetes mellitus, and tobacco use. Of these risk factors for heart failure, management of hypertension is the most important. Early work recognized the benefits of diuretics for hypertension treatment in preventing heart failure.[13,14] Recent data from the Systolic Blood Pressure Intervention Trial reinforcing this management strategy showed that intensive blood pressure control in those at higher cardiovascular disease risk treated with multiple agents to a goal systolic blood pressure ≤ 120 mm Hg led to a reduction in the composite primary outcome in nondiabetic, elderly patients and was primarily driven by a 37% reduction in the risk for nonfatal heart failure.[15] Replication of these results in younger populations would further establish effective hypertension management as a reasonable goal for stage A heart failure.

With the accumulation of risk factors for heart failure that could modify myocardial substrate, early use of noninvasive imaging, such as echocardiography, can help establish stage B heart failure, even before symptom development so that steps can be taken to ameliorate progression of disease and reduce mortality. Echocardiography in this case is commonly used to assess left ventricular dimensions, left ventricular hypertrophy, and calculation of ejection fraction. In the post–acute coronary syndrome or myocardial infarction setting, and left ventricular ejection fraction ≤40%, the Survival and Ventricular Enlargement and Carvedilol Post-Infarct Survival Control in Left Ventricular Dysfunction trials showed relative reductions in mortality by 19% and 23% in individuals treated with captopril and carvedilol, respectively, versus placebo.[16,17] These studies paved the way for angiotensin-converting enzyme inhibitors (ACEI; angiotensin receptor blockers [ARB] if not tolerated), and evidence-based beta-blockers to be formally recommended for stage B heart failure in the post–myocardial infarction setting according to the 2013 guidelines.[2] In the absence of history of myocardial infarction, the Studies of Left Ventricular Dysfunction (SOLVD) investigators established the use of ACEI in asymptomatic left ventricular dysfunction to reduce progression to symptomatic heart failure and related heart failure admissions.[18] Nonetheless, continued blood pressure management is vital in the setting of structural heart abnormalities to prevent progression to symptomatic heart failure.

Biomarker Screening for Early Intervention and the Prevention of Heart Failure

Echocardiography can be used in concert with biomarkers to better guide therapy in asymptomatic stages A and B heart failure. Brain natriuretic peptide (BNP) or its aminoterminal cleavage equivalent (NT-proBNP) are released from cardiac myocytes in response to myocardial stretch and are common biomarkers that are used as reflections of clinical heart failure. In the absence of overt heart failure symptoms reported by patients or signs detected on examination, the Screening to Prevent Heart Failure study showed that BNP elevation >50 pg/mL can be used to trigger additional evaluation in those with stage A and stage B heart failure presenting with hypertension, hyperlipidemia, obesity, vascular disease, diabetes mellitus, arrhythmia, and moderate to severe valvular dysfunction, resulting in earlier implementation of renin-angiotensin-aldosterone system (RAAS) blockade. The end result was a 35% lesser odds for major cardiovascular events as well as a reduction in heart failure–related emergency room visits.[19] Similarly, it has been shown that up-titrating RAAS and beta-receptor blockade in diabetics with no known cardiac disease until baseline elevated NT-proBNP greater than 125 pg/mL was reduced by 50% leads to significant reductions in hospitalization or death due to cardiac disease at 2 years compared with placebo.[20]

Implantable Cardiac Defibrillators in Asymptomatic Left Ventricular Dysfunction due to Ischemic Heart Disease

Despite the proven ability of RAAS and beta-receptor blockade to reduce risk for progression of heart failure and death in individuals with left ventricular dysfunction and due to ischemic heart disease, there exists a persistent risk for sudden death with left ventricular ejection fraction ≤30%. The Multicenter Automatic Defibrillator Implantation Trial II found that use of implantable cardiac defibrillators (ICD) in this population was

associated with 12% reduction in all-cause mortality at 1 year and 28% reduction in all-cause mortality at 2 and 3 years in NYHA Functional Class I-III heart failure.[21] Subgroup analyses showed that this effect remained for NYHA functional class I participants in isolation, with more than 30% reduction in the hazard for all-cause death during the trial duration. In light of this, ICD therapy is recommended for even asymptomatic stage B heart failure in individuals treated with guideline-directed medical therapy and who have persistent left ventricular ejection fraction ≤30% more than 40 days post–myocardial infarction.[21]

STAGE C HEART FAILURE
Lifestyle, Diet, and Activity as Therapies for Symptomatic Heart Failure

Management of stage C heart failure requires a holistic approach beyond pharmaceutical therapy. It is imperative that patients make necessary adjustments to their lifestyles and engage in their own care by monitoring their own symptoms, monitoring their weight, restricting sodium intake, adhering with their medications, and making every effort to remain physically active.[2] In the Heart Failure: A Controlled Trial Investigating Outcomes of Exercise Training study of HFrEF patients with nonischemic and ischemic causes, adjusted analyses showed a 9% and 15% reduction in the hazards for all-cause mortality or hospitalization and cardiovascular mortality or heart failure hospitalization with aerobic exercise training compared with usual care.[22]

Health Disparities in Heart Failure as a Function of Race, Ethnicity, and Gender

Minorities and women have traditionally been underrepresented in heart failure clinical trials. Available data suggest that African Americans, Hispanic Americans, and women with HFrEF may be undertreated with evidence-based and tailored therapy, including isosorbide dinitrate and hydralazine for African Americans and device therapy for primary prevention of sudden cardiac death among minorities and women.[23,24] Recognition of these disparities in care is important for the equitable management of heart failure in various populations.

Evidence-Based Medical Therapy for Heart Failure with Reduced Ejection Fraction

The Cooperative North Scandinavian Enalapril Survival Study heralded in the era of guideline-directed medical therapy for HFrEF with the discovery of a mortality benefit for enalapril at 6 months compared with placebo in NYHA functional class IV patients, a finding that later expanded to all symptom classes of heart failure in the SOLVD trial over a span of 41 months.[25,26] More than 10 years later, in patients unable to tolerate ACEI, ARBs were shown to be an alternative for RAAS blockade in the Valsartan Heart Failure Trial, and Candesartan in Heart Failure-Assessment of Reduction in Mortality and Morbidity (CHARM)-Alternative study yielded significant reductions in the composite endpoints.[27,28] Standard guideline-directed medical therapy for HFrEF unequivocally includes evidence-based beta-blockers: carvedilol in the US Carvedilol Study in 1996; metoprolol succinate in the Metoprolol CR/XL Randomised Intervention Trial in Congestive Heart Failure trial; and bisoprolol in the Cardiac Insufficiency Bisoprolol Study II in 1999 all generated striking survival data.[29-31] Collectively, these data reveal that among HFrEF patients, the number needed to treat to prevent one death due to any reason over 1 year is 77 and 28 for ACEI/ARB and beta-blockers, respectively (**Table 1**).[32] Those with congestive symptoms should receive diuretics in addition to ACEI/ARBs and beta-blockers at a minimum to ameliorate heart failure symptoms.[2]

Further therapy on top of background ACEI/ARB and beta-blockers for HFrEF is dictated by patient phenotypes, primarily exercise tolerance, and African American race.[2] In patients with residual NYHA functional class II-IV symptoms and reduced exercise tolerance, the Randomized Aldactone Evaluation Study and the Eplerenone in Mild Patients Hospitalization and Survival Study in Heart Failure trials paved the way for mineralocorticoid receptor antagonists (MRA), namely spironolactone and eplerenone, to become part of standard HFrEF therapy, with only 18 individuals needing to be treated to prevent 1 death over the span of a year (see **Table 1**).[32-34]

The African American Heart Failure Trial (A-HeFT) of 2004 represented a departure from traditional heart failure trials that included a heterogeneous group of participants and focused on individuals who self-identified as black.[35] In doing so, the investigators opened the door for personalized therapy for HFrEF (possibly based on phenotypic, genetic, or biomarker profiles still under investigation) and also sought to address disparities in heart failure care. The results are undeniable in that use of fixed-dose combinations of isosorbide dinitrate and hydralazine in addition to background evidenced-based medical therapy resulted in a 43% relative risk reduction for all-cause mortality and a number needed to treat of only 21 to prevent 1 death compared with placebo over 1 year among African Americans (see **Table 1**).[32,35] This latter effect nearly equals the mortality benefit of MRA therapy in HFrEF.[32] In patients who are intolerant of ACEI and ARBs due to hypotension, angioedema, hyperkalemia, or renal insufficiency, isosorbide dinitrate and hydralazine are also indicated for the management of stage C HFrEF to reduce morbidity and mortality, although the certainty of treatment effect and level of evidence are much lower.[2] Most importantly, based on the genetic substudy of the A-HeFT trial, homozygotes for a polymorphism in the guanine nucleotide-binding proteins beta-3 subunit may

Table 1
Demonstrated benefits of evidence-based therapies for patient with heart failure and reduced ejection fraction

Evidence-Based Medical Therapy	Relative Risk Reduction in All-Cause Mortality in Pivotal Randomized Control Trials	NNT to Prevent All-Cause Mortality over Time	NNT for All-Cause Mortality Standardized to 1 y
ACEI/ARB	17	22 over 42 mo	77
ARNI[a]	16	36 over 27 mo	80
Beta-blocker	34	28 over 12 mo	28
MRA	30	9 over 24 mo	18
Hydralazine/nitrate	43	25 over 10 mo	21
CRT	36	12 over 24 mo	24
ICD	23	14 over 60 mo	70

Abbreviations: CRT, cardiac resynchronization therapy; NNT, number needed to treat.
   [a] Benefit of ARNI therapy incremental to that achieved with ACEI therapy. For the other medication classes shown, the benefits shown are based on comparisons to placebo therapy.
   Adapted from Fonarow GC, Hernandez AF, Solomon SD, et al. Potential mortality reduction with optimal implementation of angiotensin receptor neprilysin inhibitor therapy in heart failure. JAMA Cardiol 2016;1(6):716; with permission.

have an enhanced response to fixed-dose combinations of isosorbide dinitrate and hydralazine. The benefit of genetic characterization is now being prospectively examined in the Genetic Risk Assessment of Heart Failure in African Americans study and may establish a path forward for future genetically tailored treatments for heart failure.[36]

Newer Medical Therapies for Heart Failure with Reduced Ejection Fraction

A 2016 focused update of the American College of Cardiology (ACC)/AHA/Heart Failure Society of America (HFSA) heart failure guidelines incorporated the results of the Prospective Comparison of ARNI (angiotensin receptor–neprilysin inhibitors) and ACEI to Determine Impact on Global Mortality and Morbidity in Heart Failure (PARADIGM-HF) and the Systolic Heart Failure Treatment with the I$_f$ inhibitor Ivabradine Trial (SHIFT) trials examining the effects of valsartan/sacubitril, an ARNI, and ivabradine, a sinoatrial node modulator, respectively, for the management of chronic heart failure.[37–39]

The PARADIGM-HF trial showed that in adult symptomatic heart failure patients with left ventricular ejection fraction ≤35% and serum natriuretic peptide elevation, valsartan/sacubitril was associated with a 20% reduction in the primary endpoint of death from cardiovascular causes or admission for heart failure. The number needed to treat was 80 to reduce death from any cause compared with doses of enalapril previously shown to reduce mortality (see **Table 1**).[26,32,37,40] As a result, patients with stage C, NYHA functional class II and II heart failure, who tolerate ACEI or ARB with an adequate blood pressure are recommended to switch to valsartan/sacubitril instead of ACEI to further reduce morbidity and mortality from heart failure.[8]

Ivabradine, thought to modulate heart rate via I$_f$ channels in the sinoatrial node with no effects on blood pressure, was effective in the SHIFT trial in reducing heart failure hospitalizations by 26% compared with placebo in patients with left ventricular ejection fraction ≤35% and NYHA class II-IV symptoms, in sinus rhythm and a resting heart rate greater than 70 beats per minute despite already being on maximally tolerated doses of beta-blockers.[38] These effects are noted across various comorbidity burdens and thus represent a novel treatment opportunity to reduce heart failure morbidity.[8,39]

Diagnostic and Therapeutic Devices for Heart Failure

Despite guideline-directed medical therapy improving heart failure mortality, hospitalization for heart failure comprises a large portion of the morbidity associated with heart failure. Efforts to reduce heart failure–related emergency room visits and admissions have prompted a search for reliable predictors of impending need for hospitalization. Telemonitoring, home weight management, left atrial monitoring, and impedance monitoring via implantable devices have all been evaluated with no clear evidence of benefit. Recently, a proprietary system, CardioMEMS device (St. Jude Medical), that assesses ambulatory pulmonary artery pressure monitoring (as a surrogate for left ventricular end-diastolic pressure) has demonstrated evidence of benefit. The Cardio-MEMS Heart Sensor Allows Monitoring of Pressure to Improve Outcomes in NYHA Class III Heart Failure Patients (CHAMPION) trial in 2011 showed that in adults with NYHA functional class III heart failure, either HFrEF or HFpEF and a prior history of heart failure hospitalization, a strategy that orchestrated treatment according to information obtained from ambulatory pulmonary artery pressure monitoring, led to 28% and 37% lower incidence of heart failure hospitalizations after 6 and 15 months of follow-up, respectively.[41] More recently, further evaluation of individuals with HFpEF in the CHAMPION study was notable for 50% relative risk reduction for heart failure hospitalization when receiving pulmonary artery pressure monitoring guided therapy versus routine symptom and physical examination–based management.[42] Among Medicare-eligible patients, all-cause 30-day readmissions were reduced by 58% in patients receiving CardioMEMS-guided ambulatory care.[43] Confirmatory studies are pending, and identification of the best patient to benefit from this new technology remains an unanswered question, but especially for those patients with HFpEF, this technology holds promise.

A Contemporary Approach to Heart Failure with Preserved Ejection Fraction

Currently, the 2013 ACCF/AHA guidelines recommend optimizing blood pressure control and using diuretics to manage heart failure morbidity for HFpEF.[2] Neurohormonal antagonists have been deemed unsuccessful in demonstrating mortality benefits for HFpEF, unlike HFrEF. Therapy for HFpEF needs to be followed according to the concomitant other comorbidities that are present. There may also be certain patients with HFpEF who might benefit from aldosterone antagonists. Even though the Treatment of Preserved Cardiac Function Heart Failure with an Aldosterone Antagonist (TOPCAT) trial had negative results, subsequent post hoc analyses have identified important variances in the data that may be of clinical significance. Results from Russia and the Democratic Republic of Georgia, both regions having contributed considerable numbers of patients to TOPCAT, have been questioned, given the absence of any evidence of a drug therapy effect and the very low event rates in the placebo arm. A prespecified subgroup trial analysis found that spironolactone (vs placebo) resulted in a significant 18% reduction in the composite primary outcome for the risk of cardiovascular death, aborted cardiac arrest, and heart failure hospitalization among HFpEF patients within the Americas who were likely to be biomarker positive and have a prior history of HF hospitalization.[44] Furthermore, the risk of cardiovascular death was reduced by 26%, and the risk of heart failure hospitalizations was reduced by 18%.[44]

Yusuf and colleagues[45] in the CHARM-Preserved trial showed that candesartan, versus placebo, resulted in a 16% reduction in the risk of heart failure hospitalizations. In addition, Cleland and colleagues,[46] in the Perindopril in Elderly People with Chronic Heart Failure trial, exhibited a significant improvement in 6-minute walk distance among HFpEF patients randomized to perindopril as opposed to placebo. These potential benefits of ACEI, ARBs, and MRA for HFpEF should not be discounted, but more precision regarding which patient and under which conditions treatment should be implemented is required.

Recognizing the fairly heterogeneous makeup up HFpEF, Shah and colleagues[47] have recently proposed phenotype-specific characterization of HFpEF. In this regard, treatment may be tailored depending on a constellation of phenotypic and comorbidity clusters (**Table 2**).

Current investigational targets for HFpEF management include ameliorating myocardial hypertrophy and stiffness via nitric oxide and cyclic guanosine monophosphate (cGMP) pathways. The Soluble Guanylate Cyclase Stimulator in Heart Failure Studies-Preserved trial is a phase 2b examining the safety and efficacy of the oral agent vericiguat in HFpEF by increasing cGMP and downstream nitric oxide bioavailability.[47,48] Furthermore, a phase 3, multicenter study examining whether the benefits of valsartan/sacubitril can be extended from HFrEF to HFpEF is underway. It is thought that RAAS blockade and neprilysin inhibition will increase cGMP and reduce cardiomyocyte hypertrophy, stiffness, interstitial fibrosis, and endothelial dysfunction while also improving skeletal muscle and renal function. How this approach will influence clinical endpoints is not yet clear.[47,49]

STAGE D HEART FAILURE

Stage D heart failure represents refractory heart failure that may require advanced therapeutics beyond guideline-directed medical therapy, including mechanical support, cardiac transplantation, and in certain scenarios, end-of-life care.[9] As per the 2013 ACCF/AHA guidelines, cardiac inotropic support is recommended for cardiogenic shock while deciding what type of further treatment strategy should be used, as a bridge to transplant or durable mechanical support, as even as part of a long-term palliative treatment strategy.[2]

Palliative Care and Hospice Therapy

Imperative to the management of stage D heart failure are discussions on palliative and hospice care with patients. The HFSA's 2015 statement on stage D heart failure emphasizes that such discussions are needed to better understand whether patients would rather focus on quality or quantity of life.[50] If the former is preferred, heart failure care teams can then arrange care based on such measures. The Centers for Medicare and Medicaid Services require that approval for mechanical support and cardiac transplantation necessitates involving palliative care and hospice care specialists in care discussions so that patients can pursue treatment decisions best suited to their preferences via shared decision making.[50] Nonetheless, palliative and hospice care appears to be underutilized in the remaining months of life in many patients with refractory heart failure, whereby less than 10% of those with the highest decile of mortality risk receive such care in the AHA's Get With the Guidelines program.[51] Such statistics can be ameliorated by adopting frameworks set forth in the HFSA consensus statement on end-of-life care, including how to even initiate discussions on palliative and hospice care.[52]

Ventricular Replacement

As mentioned above, using shared decision making, patients should be evaluated for advanced therapies, including cardiac transplantation and durable mechanical support, as destination therapy or a bridge to cardiac transplantation.

Transplant

Cardiac transplantation remains the gold standard for treating stage D heart failure with roughly 6300 heart transplants being performed each year worldwide.[2,53] Advancements in immunosuppressive therapy, namely the use of calcineurin inhibitors (tacrolimus or cyclosporine) and antiproliferative agents (mycophenolate mofetil or azathioprine) as the cornerstone of maintenance therapy, have

Table 2

Phenotype-specific HFpEF treatment strategy using a matrix of predisposition phenotypes and clinical presentation phenotypes

HFpEF Clinical Presentation Phenotypes

HFpEF Predisposition Phenotypes	Lung Congestion	+ Chronotropic Incompetence	+ Pulmonary Hypertension (CpcPH)	+ Skeletal Muscle Weakness	+ Atrial Fibrillation
Overweight/ obesity/ metabolic syndrome/ type 2 DM	• **Diuretics (loop diuretic in DM)** • **Caloric restriction** • Statins • Inorganic nitrite/nitrate • Sacubitril • Spironolactone	+Rate adaptive atrial pacing	+Pulmonary vasodilators (eg, PDE5I)	+Exercise training program	+Cardioversion +Rate control +**Anticoagulation**
+ Arterial hypertension	+ACEI/ARB	+ACEI/ARB +Rate adaptive atrial pacing	+ACEI/ARB +Pulmonary vasodilators (eg, PDE5I)	+ACEI/ARB +**Exercise training program**	+ACEI/ARB +Cardioversion +Rate control +**Anticoagulation**
+ Renal dysfunction	+Ultrafiltration if needed	+Ultrafiltration if needed +Rate adaptive atrial pacing	+Ultrafiltration if needed +Pulmonary vasodilators (eg, PDE5I)	+Ultrafiltration if needed +**Exercise training program**	+Ultrafiltration if needed +Cardioversion +Rate control +**Anticoagulation**
+ CAD	+ACEI +Revascularization	+ACEI +Revascularization +Rate adaptive atrial pacing	+ACEI +Revascularization +Pulmonary vasodilators (eg, PDE5I)	+ACEI +Revascularization +**Exercise training program**	+ACEI +Revascularization +Cardioversion +Rate control +**Anticoagulation**

Abbreviations: CAD, coronary artery disease; CpcPH, combined precapillary and postcapillary pulmonary hypertension; DM, diabetes mellitus; PDE5I, phosphodiesterase-5 inhibitor.

Adapted from Shah SJ, Kitzman DW, Borlaug BA, et al. Phenotype-specific treatment of heart failure with preserved ejection fraction. Circulation 2016;134(1):76; with permission.

resulted in median survival exceeding 80% and 70% at 1 and 5 years, respectively, since 2002.[53] Listing criteria for heart transplantation have been recently updated by the International Society for Heart and Lung Transplantation.[54] Notable changes include liberalizing recommended cutoffs for renal impairment and obesity ahead of cardiac transplant, greater weight on frailty and psychosocial assessments, considering higher prioritization for highly sensitized patients, and retransplantation for individuals with significant coronary allograft vasculopathy despite no other signs of rejection.[54]

Left ventricular assist devices

Short-term percutaneous and surgical mechanical support, including intra-aortic balloon pumps, Impella® (Abiomed) devices, and extracorporeal membrane oxygenation, can be used as bridges to myocardial recovery or even to a decision as to whether a patient would be a suitable candidate for more durable mechanical support or cardiac transplantation.[2] Data from the Nationwide Inpatient Sample, Healthcare Cost, and Utilization Project show a 101% increase in the use of nonpercutaneous mechanical support and a 1511% increase in the use of percutaneous mechanical support between 2007 and 2011 owing to lower costs, earlier implementation, and improved mortality with such devices.[55]

The HeartMate II™ (St. Jude Corporation) axial flow pump and the HVAD® (HeartWare) centrifugal pump are approved as durable, implantable left ventricular assist devices (LVAD) as bridges to cardiac transplant. In such situations, these devices help alleviate pulmonary hypertension and allow patients to address such factors as obesity and tobacco use that would otherwise preclude cardiac transplant.[2,56,57]

The Randomized Evaluation of Mechanical Assistance for the Treatment of Congestive Heart Failure trial established the use of permanent, implantable left ventricular assist devices as an alternative management strategy for individuals with stage D heart failure ineligible for cardiac transplantation with a significant 48% reduction in death from any cause and significant improvements in quality of life, including depression scores and NYHA functional class.[58] Currently the HeartMate II™ device is approved for destination therapy. Recently, a comparison study between the HeartMate 3™ (St. Jude Corporation) pulsatile LVAD and the HeartMate II™ continuous flow LVAD was completed. Early follow-up data at six months are consistent with a lesser need for pump re-operation and virtually zero cases of pump thrombosis. If longer-term data validate

clinical improvements and device durability, this could reflect a breakthrough in LVAD technology.[59] Active areas of investigation include the use of durable left ventricular assist devices to facilitate myocardial recovery, and the efficacy of a lateral thoracotomy versus conventional median sternotomy on survival, adverse events, and perioperative outcomes for the HVAD® system.[60,61]

FUTURE THERAPEUTIC CONSIDERATIONS

Although neurohormonal therapy is the mainstay of medical management of HFrEF, the need for mechanical support or cardiac transplantation in patients with stage D heart failure necessitates a search for other therapies that can ideally promote myocardial recovery and obviate ventricular replacement strategies. Regenerative therapy via stem cells or gene transfer may be the next frontier for heart failure management. Multiple trials since 2002 have looked at the effects of bone marrow–derived mononuclear cells and mesenchymal stem cells in ischemic/infarcted hearts on myocardial recovery, but progress has been hindered by mixed results often at translational stages.[62] Nonetheless, Chong and colleagues[63] recently reported that human embryonic stem cell–derived cardiomyocytes can be produced on a clinical scale, cryopreserved, and delivered directly to the myocardium to regenerate hearts in non–human primates. Despite a prior focus on ischemic heart disease and left ventricular dysfunction, active research is also being undertaken to assess mesenchymal stem cells for dilated, nonischemic cardiomyopathy.[64] Last, Hammond and colleagues[65] recently reported that intracoronary gene transfer of adenylyl cyclase 6 (which catalyzes adenosine triphosphate to cyclic adenosine monophosphate) in a phase 2 trial led to a significant 6% increase in left ventricular function at 4 weeks versus placebo and a nonsignificant trend toward less heart failure admissions during the study period.

SUMMARY

Incident heart failure and heart failure admissions are now decreasing while the prevalence and costs remain high. The burden of mortality is also compelling, but earlier and better detection of heart failure and the availability and implementation of evidence-based therapy to reduce morbidity and mortality for HFrEF remain the target in contemporary practice. Ventricular replacement with durable mechanical support or heart transplantation is increasingly being used for end-stage HFrEF.

There is a growing burden of HFpEF, for which no available therapies are approved yet to reduce mortality. Future heart failure clinical trials will need to focus on reducing HFpEF morbidity and mortality. It is critical to address the morbidity associated with an increasing number of years lived with heart failure as the annual economic cost of heart failure care, currently estimated at $30.7 billion, is expected to more than double by 2030. The future of heart failure care may finally encompass true personalized medicine driven by genomics and other biomarkers while definitive therapy for heart failure may encompass biological ventricular replacement strategies using cell or gene based regenerative therapies.

REFERENCES

1. Mozaffarian D, Benjamin EJ, Go AS, et al. Heart disease and stroke statistics—2016 update: a report from the American Heart Association. Circulation 2016;133(4):e38–360.
2. Yancy CW, Jessup M, Bozkurt B, et al. 2013 ACCF/AHA guideline for the management of heart failure: a report of the American College of Cardiology Foundation/American Heart Association Task Force on Practice guidelines. J Am Coll Cardiol 2013;62(16): e147–239.
3. Kalogeropoulos AP, Fonarow GC, Georgiopoulou V, et al. Characteristics and outcomes of adult outpatients with heart failure and improved or recovered ejection fraction. JAMA Cardiol 2016;1(5):510–8.
4. Wilcox JE, Yancy CW. Heart failure—a new phenotype emerges. JAMA Cardiol 2016;1(5):507–9.
5. Gerber Y, Weston SA, Redfield MM, et al. A contemporary appraisal of the heart failure epidemic in Olmsted County, Minnesota, 2000 to 2010. JAMA Intern Med 2015;175(6):996–1004.
6. Bergethon KE, Ju C, DeVore AD, et al. Trends in 30-day readmission rates for patients hospitalized with heart failure: findings from the Get With the Guidelines-Heart Failure Registry. Circ Heart Fail 2016;9(6):e002594.
7. Krumholz HM, Normand S-LT, Wang Y. Trends in hospitalizations and outcomes for acute cardiovascular disease and stroke, 1999-2011. Circulation 2014;130(12):966–75.
8. Yancy CW, Jessup M, Bozkurt B, et al. 2016 ACC/AHA/HFSA focused update on new pharmacological therapy for heart failure: an update of the 2013 ACCF/AHA guideline for the management of heart failure: a report of the American College of Cardiology/American Heart Association Task Force on Clinical Practice guidelines and the Heart Failure Society of America. J Am Coll Cardiol 2016;68(13):1476–88.
9. Hunt SA, Abraham WT, Chin MH, et al. 2009 focused update incorporated into the ACC/AHA 2005 guidelines for the diagnosis and management of heart failure in adults a report of the American College of Cardiology Foundation/American Heart Association Task Force on Practice Guidelines developed in Collaboration with the International Society for Heart and Lung Transplantation. J Am Coll Cardiol 2009;53(15):e1–90.
10. Dolgin M. Nomenclature and criteria for diagnosis of diseases of the heart and great vessels. Boston (MA): Little, Brown Medical Division; 1994.
11. Go AS, Bauman MA, Coleman King SM, et al. An effective approach to high blood pressure control: a science advisory from the American Heart Association, the American College of Cardiology, and the Centers for Disease Control and Prevention. J Am Coll Cardiol 2014;63(12):1230–8.
12. Stone NJ, Robinson JG, Lichtenstein AH, et al. 2013 ACC/AHA guideline on the treatment of blood cholesterol to reduce atherosclerotic cardiovascular risk in adults: a report of the American College of Cardiology/American Heart Association Task Force on Practice Guidelines. J Am Coll Cardiol 2014; 63(25 Pt B):2889–934.
13. Kostis JB, Davis BR, Cutler J, et al. Prevention of heart failure by antihypertensive drug treatment in older persons with isolated systolic hypertension. SHEP Cooperative Research Group. JAMA 1997; 278(3):212–6.
14. Sciarretta S, Palano F, Tocci G, et al. Antihypertensive treatment and development of heart failure in hypertension: a Bayesian network meta-analysis of studies in patients with hypertension and high cardiovascular risk. Arch Intern Med 2011;171(5):384–94.
15. Williamson JD, Supiano MA, Applegate WB, et al. Intensive vs standard blood pressure control and cardiovascular disease outcomes in adults aged ≥75 years: a randomized clinical trial. JAMA 2016; 315(24):2673–82.
16. Pfeffer MA, Braunwald E, Moyé LA, et al. Effect of captopril on mortality and morbidity in patients with left ventricular dysfunction after myocardial infarction. Results of the survival and ventricular enlargement trial. The SAVE Investigators. N Engl J Med 1992;327(10):669–77.
17. Dargie HJ. Effect of carvedilol on outcome after myocardial infarction in patients with left-ventricular dysfunction: the CAPRICORN randomised trial. Lancet 2001;357(9266):1385–90.
18. Effect of enalapril on mortality and the development of heart failure in asymptomatic patients with reduced left ventricular ejection fractions. The SOLVD Investigators. N Engl J Med 1992;327(10): 685–91.
19. Ledwidge M, Gallagher J, Conlon C, et al. Natriuretic peptide-based screening and collaborative care for heart failure: the STOP-HF randomized trial. JAMA 2013;310(1):66–74.

20. Huelsmann M, Neuhold S, Resl M, et al. PONTIAC (NT-proBNP selected prevention of cardiac events in a population of diabetic patients without a history of cardiac disease): a prospective randomized controlled trial. J Am Coll Cardiol 2013;62(15): 1365–72.

21. Moss AJ, Zareba W, Hall WJ, et al. Prophylactic implantation of a defibrillator in patients with myocardial infarction and reduced ejection fraction. N Engl J Med 2002;346(12):877–83.

22. O'Connor CM, Whellan DJ, Lee KL, et al. Efficacy and safety of exercise training in patients with chronic heart failure: HF-ACTION randomized controlled trial. JAMA 2009;301(14):1439–50.

23. Khazanie P, Liang L, Curtis LH, et al. Clinical effectiveness of hydralazine-isosorbide dinitrate therapy in patients with heart failure and reduced ejection fraction: findings from the Get With the Guidelines-Heart Failure Registry. Circ Heart Fail 2016;9(2): e002444.

24. Hess PL, Hernandez AF, Bhatt DL, et al. Sex and race/ethnicity differences in implantable cardioverter-defibrillator counseling and use among patients hospitalized with heart failure: findings from the Get With the Guidelines-Heart Failure Program. Circulation 2016;134(7):517–26.

25. Effects of enalapril on mortality in severe congestive heart failure. Results of the Cooperative North Scandinavian enalapril survival study (CONSENSUS). The CONSENSUS trial study group. N Engl J Med 1987;316(23):1429–35.

26. Effect of enalapril on survival in patients with reduced left ventricular ejection fractions and congestive heart failure. The SOLVD Investigators. N Engl J Med 1991;325(5):293–302.

27. Cohn JN, Tognoni G. Valsartan Heart Failure Trial Investigators. A randomized trial of the angiotensin-receptor blocker valsartan in chronic heart failure. N Engl J Med 2001;345(23):1667–75.

28. Granger CB, McMurray JJV, Yusuf S, et al. Effects of candesartan in patients with chronic heart failure and reduced left-ventricular systolic function intolerant to angiotensin-converting-enzyme inhibitors: the CHARM-Alternative trial. Lancet 2003;362(9386): 772–6.

29. Packer M, Bristow MR, Cohn JN, et al. The effect of carvedilol on morbidity and mortality in patients with chronic heart failure. U.S. Carvedilol Heart Failure Study Group. N Engl J Med 1996;334(21):1349–55.

30. Effect of metoprolol CR/XL in chronic heart failure: metoprolol CR/XL randomised intervention trial in congestive heart failure (MERIT-HF). Lancet 1999; 353(9169):2001–7.

31. The cardiac insufficiency bisoprolol study II (CIBIS-II): a randomised trial. Lancet 1999;353(9146):9–13.

32. Fonarow GC, Hernandez AF, Solomon SD, et al. Potential mortality reduction with optimal implementation of angiotensin receptor neprilysin inhibitor therapy in heart failure. JAMA Cardiol 2016;1(6):714–7.

33. Pitt B, Zannad F, Remme WJ, et al. The effect of spironolactone on morbidity and mortality in patients with severe heart failure. Randomized Aldactone Evaluation Study Investigators. N Engl J Med 1999;341(10):709–17.

34. Zannad F, McMurray JJV, Krum H, et al. Eplerenone in patients with systolic heart failure and mild symptoms. N Engl J Med 2011;364(1):11–21.

35. Taylor AL, Ziesche S, Yancy C, et al. Combination of isosorbide dinitrate and hydralazine in blacks with heart failure. N Engl J Med 2004;351(20):2049–57.

36. McNamara DM, Taylor AL, Tam SW, et al. G-protein beta-3 subunit genotype predicts enhanced benefit of fixed-dose isosorbide dinitrate and hydralazine: results of A-HeFT. JACC Heart Fail 2014;2(6):551–7.

37. McMurray JJV, Packer M, Desai AS, et al. Angiotensin-neprilysin inhibition versus enalapril in heart failure. N Engl J Med 2014;371(11):993–1004.

38. Swedberg K, Komajda M, Böhm M, et al. Ivabradine and outcomes in chronic heart failure (SHIFT): a randomised placebo-controlled study. Lancet 2010;376(9744):875–85.

39. Böhm M, Robertson M, Ford I, et al. Influence of cardiovascular and noncardiovascular co-morbidities on outcomes and treatment effect of heart rate reduction with ivabradine in stable heart failure (from the shift trial). Am J Cardiol 2015;116(12): 1890–7.

40. Jessup M. Neprilysin inhibition–a novel therapy for heart failure. N Engl J Med 2014;371(11):1062–4.

41. Abraham WT, Adamson PB, Bourge RC, et al. Wireless pulmonary artery haemodynamic monitoring in chronic heart failure: a randomised controlled trial. Lancet 2011;377(9766):658–66.

42. Adamson PB, Abraham WT, Bourge RC, et al. Wireless pulmonary artery pressure monitoring guides management to reduce decompensation in heart failure with preserved ejection fraction. Circ Heart Fail 2014;7(6):935–44.

43. Adamson PB, Abraham WT, Stevenson LW, et al. Pulmonary artery pressure-guided heart failure management reduces 30-day readmissions. Circ Heart Fail 2016;9(6):e002600.

44. Pfeffer MA, Claggett B, Assmann SF, et al. Regional variation in patients and outcomes in the treatment of preserved cardiac function heart failure with an aldosterone antagonist (TOPCAT) trial. Circulation 2015;131(1):34–42.

45. Yusuf S, Pfeffer MA, Swedberg K, et al. Effects of candesartan in patients with chronic heart failure and preserved left-ventricular ejection fraction: the CHARM-Preserved Trial. Lancet 2003;362(9386): 777–81.

46. Cleland JGF, Tendera M, Adamus J, et al. The perindopril in elderly people with chronic heart

failure (PEP-CHF) study. Eur Heart J 2006;27(19): 2338–45.

47. Shah SJ, Kitzman DW, Borlaug BA, et al. Phenotype-specific treatment of heart failure with preserved ejection fraction. Circulation 2016;134(1):73–90.

48. Pieske B, Butler J, Filippatos G, et al. Rationale and design of the SOluble guanylate Cyclase stimulatoR in heArT failurE Studies (SOCRATES). Eur J Heart Fail 2014;16(9):1026–38.

49. Mitter SS, Shah SJ. Spironolactone for management of heart failure with preserved ejection fraction: whither to after TOPCAT? Curr Atheroscler Rep 2015;17(11):64.

50. Fang JC, Ewald GA, Allen LA, et al. Advanced (stage D) heart failure: a statement from the heart failure Society of America Guidelines Committee. J Card Fail 2015;21(6):519–34.

51. Whellan DJ, Cox M, Hernandez AF, et al. Utilization of hospice and predicted mortality risk among older patients hospitalized with heart failure: findings from GWTG-HF. J Card Fail 2012;18(6):471–7.

52. Whellan DJ, Goodlin SJ, Dickinson MG, et al. End-of-life care in patients with heart failure. J Card Fail 2014;20(2):121–34.

53. Lund LH, Edwards LB, Kucheryavaya AY, et al. The registry of the International Society for Heart and Lung Transplantation: thirty-first official adult heart transplant report–2014; focus theme: retransplantation. J Heart Lung Transplant 2014;33(10):996–1008.

54. Mehra MR, Canter CE, Hannan MM, et al. The 2016 International Society for Heart Lung Transplantation listing criteria for heart transplantation: a 10-year update. J Heart Lung Transplant 2016;35(1):1–23.

55. Stretch R, Sauer CM, Yuh DD, et al. National trends in the utilization of short-term mechanical circulatory support: incidence, outcomes, and cost analysis. J Am Coll Cardiol 2014;64(14):1407–15.

56. Alba AC, Rao V, Ross HJ, et al. Impact of fixed pulmonary hypertension on post-heart transplant outcomes in bridge-to-transplant patients. J Heart Lung Transplant 2010;29(11):1253–8.

57. Nair PK, Kormos RL, Teuteberg JJ, et al. Pulsatile left ventricular assist device support as a bridge to decision in patients with end-stage heart failure complicated by pulmonary hypertension. J Heart Lung Transplant 2010;29(2):201–8.

58. Rose EA, Gelijns AC, Moskowitz AJ, et al. Long-term use of a left ventricular assist device for end-stage heart failure. N Engl J Med 2001;345(20):1435–43.

59. Mehra MR, Naka Y, Uriel N, et al. A fully magnetically levitated circulatory pump for advanced heart failure. N Engl J Med 2017;376(5):440–50.

60. Hall JL, Fermin DR, Birks EJ, et al. Clinical, molecular, and genomic changes in response to a left ventricular assist device. J Am Coll Cardiol 2011;57(6): 641–52.

61. Kato TS, Chokshi A, Singh P, et al. Effects of continuous-flow versus pulsatile-flow left ventricular assist devices on myocardial unloading and remodeling. Circ Heart Fail 2011;4(5):546–53.

62. Gerbin KA, Murry CE. The winding road to regenerating the human heart. Cardiovasc Pathol 2015; 24(3):133–40.

63. Chong JJH, Yang X, Don CW, et al. Human embryonic-stem-cell-derived cardiomyocytes regenerate non-human primate hearts. Nature 2014; 510(7504):273–7.

64. Greene SJ, Epstein SE, Kim RJ, et al. Rationale and design of a randomized controlled trial of allogeneic mesenchymal stem cells in patients with nonischemic cardiomyopathy. J Cardiovasc Med (Hagerstown) 2015. [Epub ahead of print].

65. Hammond HK, Penny WF, Traverse JH, et al. Intracoronary gene transfer of adenylyl cyclase 6 in patients with heart failure: a randomized clinical trial. JAMA Cardiol 2016;1(2):163–71.

Special Articles

The Role of Implantable Hemodynamic Monitors to Manage Heart Failure

William T. Abraham, MD, FACP, FACC, FAHA, FESC, FRCP

KEYWORDS

- Disease management • Heart failure • Hemodynamics • Hospitalization • Left atrial pressure
- Pulmonary artery pressure • Quality of life

KEY POINTS

- Heart failure is associated with high rates of hospitalization and rehospitalization.
- Current approaches to monitoring heart failure have done little to reduce these high rates of hospitalization and rehospitalization.
- Implantable hemodynamic monitors provide direct measurements of intracardiac and pulmonary artery pressures in ambulatory patients with heart failure.
- Heart failure care guided by implantable hemodynamic monitors reduces the risk of heart failure hospitalization and improves quality of life.

INTRODUCTION

Heart failure represents a major and growing public health concern, associated with high rates of hospitalization and rehospitalization. Heart failure is the primary diagnosis in more than 1 million hospitalizations annually in the United States.[1] It is associated with the highest rate of hospital readmission compared with all other medical or surgical causes of hospitalization.[2] Approximately 25% of discharged patients are readmitted within 30 days and about 67% are readmitted within 1 year, following the index hospitalization.[2–4] Lack of improvement in health-related quality of life after discharge from the hospital is a powerful predictor of rehospitalization and mortality.[5]

Hospitalization for heart failure results in a substantial economic burden. In 2012, the US total economic burden from heart failure was estimated at $31 billion.[1] The direct costs of heart failure in the United States are estimated at $21 billion annually; of this amount, 80% of costs are from hospitalizations.[6] Without improvements in current clinical outcomes, the US total economic burden from heart failure is expected to rise to $70 billion annually by the year 2030.[1,6] Consequently, a major goal in heart failure management is to keep patients well and out of the hospital and to reduce these costs.

Unfortunately, current approaches to monitoring patients with heart failure have generally focused on insensitive noninvasive markers of heart failure clinical status and failed to improve quality of life or to reduce hospitalization rates. Worsening heart failure symptoms, changes in vital signs, and weight gain are late and unreliable markers of worsening heart failure. Implantable hemodynamic monitors, which remotely provide direct measurement of intracardiac and pulmonary artery pressures (PAP)

This article originally appeared in Heart Failure Clinics, Volume 11, Issue 2, April 2015.

Disclosures: Dr W.T. Abraham has received consulting fees from CardioMEMS for his role as Co-Principal Investigator of the CHAMPION trial and from St. Jude Medical for his role as Principal Investigator of the HOMEO-STASIS and LAPTOP-HF trials.

Division of Cardiovascular Medicine, The Ohio State University, 473 West 12th Avenue, Room 110P, Columbus, OH 43210–1252, USA

E-mail address: William.Abraham@osumc.edu

in ambulatory patients with heart failure, enable a proactive approach that shifts the focus from crisis management to stability management in patients with heart failure. This article reviews current knowledge on the role of implantable hemodynamic monitors in heart failure management.

LIMITATIONS OF CURRENT STANDARD OF CARE MONITORING IN HEART FAILURE

Noninvasive remote monitoring of patients with heart failure generally involves regularly scheduled structured telephone contact between patients and health care providers and/or the electronic transfer of physiologic data using remote access technology via electronic devices. This approach allows for the assessment of symptoms, vital signs, and daily weights, and other noninvasive parameters of interest. The efficacy of such noninvasive monitoring methods remains uncertain, although a growing body of evidence suggests that its value is limited.

Two recent large meta-analyses of randomized controlled trials and observational cohort studies suggest that remote monitoring of symptoms, vital signs, and daily weights may be beneficial for reducing death, hospitalizations, and rehospitalizations for heart failure.[7,8] In contrast, two recent large prospective randomized controlled trials challenge these findings.

In a study sponsored by the National Institutes of Health called TELE-HF, 1653 patients recently hospitalized for heart failure were randomized to undergo either remote monitoring or usual care.[9] Remote monitoring was accomplished by means of a telephone-based interactive voice-response system that collected daily information about symptoms and weight that was reviewed by clinicians, providing the opportunity for outpatient intervention to avoid hospitalization. There was no significant difference between groups in the primary end point of readmissions or death for any cause at 180 days. Hospitalizations for heart failure, the number of days in hospital, and the total number of hospitalizations were not significantly reduced by use of the remote monitoring system.

Similarly, the European randomized controlled TIM-HF trial assigned patients with heart failure with reduced left ventricular ejection fractions (LVEF) to daily remote monitoring, including an electrocardiogram, blood pressure measurement, and assessment of body weight, coupled with medical telephone support or to usual care directed by the patient's local physician.[10] After 2 years of follow-up, there was no significant difference in the primary end point of all-cause mortality or in the composite of cardiovascular death

or heart failure hospitalization between the two groups.

One reason for the failure of noninvasive remote monitoring to consistently improve clinical outcomes may be the relatively low sensitivity of changes in symptoms, vital signs, and daily weights to predict heart failure hospitalizations. For example, the sensitivity of weight change in predicting worsening heart failure events is on the order of only 10% to 20%.[11,12] In addition, weight gain and symptoms of clinical congestion (eg, worsening shortness of breath) are late manifestations of worsening heart failure. Thus, when these changes occur, the opportunity to prevent heart failure hospitalization may already be lost. Earlier markers of worsening heart failure may include autonomic adaptation and changes in intrathoracic impedance reflective of increasing lung water.[12–16] However, because clinical congestion, weight change, autonomic adaptation, and changes in intrathoracic impedance are all preceded for many days or weeks by increases in intracardiac pressure and PAP (or hemodynamic congestion), targeting pressure changes in the monitoring and management of heart failure may provide the earliest opportunity for intervention and avoidance of heart failure hospitalizations (**Fig. 1**). This is the premise supporting the use of implantable hemodynamic monitors in the management of heart failure.

IMPLANTABLE HEMODYNAMIC MONITORING

A variety of approaches to remote ambulatory monitoring of intracardiac pressure and PAP have been developed over the years. Devices targeting measurement of right ventricular pressure, PAP, and left atrial pressure (LAP) have been studied. Recently, one system for PAP monitoring received regulatory approval in the United States, ushering in a new era of implantable hemodynamic monitoring for the management of patients with heart failure.

Right Ventricular Pressure Monitors

The ability to estimate pulmonary artery end-diastolic pressure (ePAD) from the right ventricle (RV) was described in 1995.[17] Based on the observation that RV pressure at the time of pulmonary valve opening is equal to pulmonary artery diastolic pressure, RV pressure at the time of RV maximum change in pressure over time (dP/dt) was considered the ePAD and this correlated with directly measured pulmonary artery diastolic pressures at baseline, during isometric work, and during the Valsalva maneuver. This observation

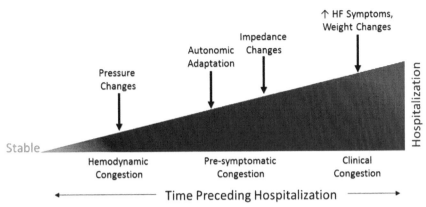

Fig. 1. Progression from stable compensated to decompensated heart failure. The earliest manifestations of worsening heart failure leading to hospitalization are increase in intracardiac pressure and PAP that occur several days to weeks before worsening symptoms and weight gain. Intermediate markers of worsening heart failure may include autonomic adaptation and changes in intrathoracic impedance reflective of increasing lung water. Changes in symptoms and daily weights occur late in this progression. HF, heart failure.

was incorporated into an implantable leaded RV pressure monitoring system, which looked similar to a single-lead permanent pacemaker, to continuously measure RV systolic and diastolic pressures, ePAD, RV dP/dt, heart rate, patient activity level, and temperature. In 32 New York Heart Association (NYHA) class II and class III patients with heart failure evaluated in an observational study of this device, RV pressures and the ePAD were shown to increase several days before worsening symptoms and heart failure hospitalization.[18] This pilot study led to the first randomized controlled trial of implantable hemodynamic monitoring for heart failure.

That study was called the Chronicle Offers Management to Patients with Advanced Signs and Symptoms of Heart Failure (COMPASS-HF) trial. COMPASS-HF randomized 274 NYHA class III and ambulatory class IV patients with heart failure to usual care alone versus usual care plus care guided by knowledge from the RV sensor system.[19] The study demonstrated a nonsignificant 21% reduction in the RV sensor group compared with the control group in the primary efficacy end point of heart failure events (hospitalizations, emergency or urgent care visits requiring intravenous therapy). COMPASS-HF was underpowered for its primary end point, and clinicians generally failed to adequately lower ePAD without target values or an algorithm to guide therapy. Thus, the hypothesis that lower pressures result in reduced rates of heart failure events was not adequately tested in this study.

However, COMPASS-HF did confirm the association of elevated PAP with increased risk of worsening heart failure events.[20] It also defined a range of pressures associated with a reduced

risk of heart failure events. Based on the 24-hour mean ePAD, pressures between 10 and 24 mm Hg were associated with a significantly lower risk of heart failure events compared with pressures of 25 mm Hg or higher. These observations suggest that lowering pressures into the normal or near normal range, even in the absence of heart failure symptoms, might reduce the risk of heart failure hospitalizations. This hypothesis was carried forward to subsequent studies of implantable hemodynamic monitors in heart failure.

Pulmonary Artery Pressure Monitors

A novel wireless PAP measurement system was recently evaluated in the CardioMEMS Heart Sensor Allows Monitoring of Pressure to Improve Outcomes in NYHA Class III Heart Failure Patients (CHAMPION) trial.[21,22] This system was previously shown to be safe and accurate in a pilot study.[23] The PAP sensor is comprised of a coil and a pressure-sensitive capacitor encased in a capsule (**Fig. 2**A). It has no battery, so there is nothing to run out or to be replaced. It is implanted into a branch of the pulmonary artery during right heart catheterization, using a specialized delivery system. Pressure applied to the sensor causes deflections of the pressure-sensitive surface, resulting in a characteristic shift in the resonant frequency. Electromagnetic coupling is achieved by an external antenna, which is held against the patient's body or embedded in a pillow (see **Fig. 2**B). The antenna provides power to the device, continuously measuring its resonant frequency, which is then converted to a pressure waveform. Pressure data are then transmitted wirelessly to a secure Web site, where clinicians

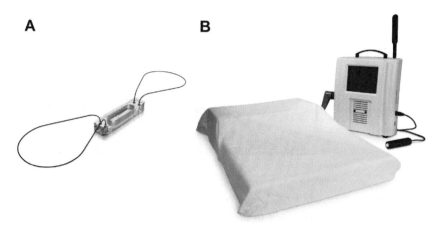

Fig. 2. PAP measurement system. (*A*) The PAP MEMS-based sensor. (*B*) An antenna embedded in a pillow simultaneously powers and interrogates the sensor using radiofrequency. (*Courtesy of* St. Jude Medical, St Paul, MN; with permission.)

can inspect discrete data or pressure trends graphed longitudinally over time.

The CHAMPION trial randomized 550 NYHA class III patients with heart failure, regardless of LVEF, to a treatment group (N = 270) where clinicians had access to daily PAP measurements and used them, in addition to standard of care heart failure monitoring, to manage patients versus a control group (N = 280) where clinicians had no access to daily PAP measurements and managed patients using standard of care heart failure monitoring alone. The CHAMPION trial differed from prior studies of implantable hemodynamic monitors in that specific pressure targets and treatment algorithms were mandated by protocol to ensure adequate testing of the hypothesis. Protocol-specified pressure goals were pulmonary artery systolic pressure 15 to 35 mm Hg, pulmonary artery diastolic pressure 8 to 20 mm Hg, and pulmonary artery mean pressure 10 to 25 mm Hg. Patients were consider hypervolemic and at-risk for heart failure hospitalization if their pressures were higher than these ranges. The goal in these patients was to lower PAP to within the target ranges, unless limited by an untoward clinical effect of PAP lowering (eg, symptomatic hypotension, clinically meaningful worsening of renal function). Protocol-guided responses to hypervolemia included initiation or intensification of diuretics, initiation or intensification of long-acting nitrates, and initiation or intensification of education regarding dietary salt and fluid restrictions. An example of PAP-guided heart failure therapy in a hypervolemic patient is shown in **Fig. 3**.

The primary end point of the CHAMPION trial was the rate of heart failure hospitalizations over 6 months. However, all patients were kept in their

randomized, single-blind study assignment until the last patient reached 6 months of follow-up, so that the long-term effectiveness of the approach could be evaluated.

There were few device-related or system-related complications and no pressure sensor failures in the CHAMPION trial. Freedom from device-related or system-related complications was 98.6%, and overall freedom from pressure-sensor failures was 100%. During the first 6 months following randomization, significantly fewer heart failure hospitalizations occurred in the treatment group (83 hospitalizations) compared with the control group (120 hospitalizations), yielding a relative risk reduction of 28% (*P*<.00002). During the entire single-blinded follow-up period averaging more than 15 months, the treatment group demonstrated a 37% relative risk reduction in heart failure hospitalizations compared with the control group. Most pressure-based medication changes involved diuretics and long-acting nitrates. Heart failure management guided by daily PAP measurement also resulted in significant PAP reduction, a decrease in the proportion of patients hospitalized for heart failure, an increase in the number of days alive and out of the hospital for heart failure, and an improvement in quality of life score. This first positive randomized controlled trial of implantable hemodynamic monitoring in patients with heart failure led to the regulatory approval of the PAP measurement system on May 28, 2014 (http://www.fda.gov/NewsEvents/Newsroom/PressAnnouncements/ucm399024.htm).

An important prespecified subgroup analysis of the CHAMPION trial evaluated the efficacy of PAP-guided heart failure therapy in patients with

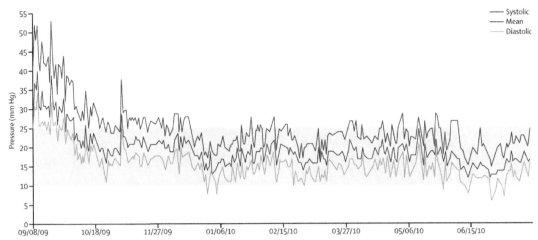

Fig. 3. Example of PAP-guided heart failure therapy from the CHAMPION trial. Pressure data uploaded to a secure Web site are used to guide pressure-based medication changes, with the goal of reducing PAP into the target range depicted by the shaded area for PA mean pressure. In this patient example, increased diuretic dosing was used to lower the initially elevated pressures into the target range and to keep it there, to reduce the risk of heart failure rehospitalization. This patient was not rehospitalized during CHAMPION trial follow-up. (*Courtesy of* St. Jude Medical, St Paul, MN; with permission.)

a preserved LVEF.[22,24] Heart failure hospitalizations were analyzed in subgroups by baseline LVEF less than 40% and 40% or greater.[22] In an additional analysis, the subgroup of patients with LVEF of 50% or greater was also analyzed.[24] Patients in the treatment group had a significant reduction in the rate of heart failure hospitalizations compared with those in the control group for preserved and reduced LVEF during 6 months (**Table 1**). Thus, PAP-guided heart failure management represents the first approach to demonstrate improved clinical outcomes in patients with heart failure with a preserved LVEF.

Another key subgroup analysis of CHAMPION trial data evaluated the utility of PAP-guided therapy in patients with heart failure with World Health Organization group II pulmonary hypertension.[25] This retrospective analysis demonstrated the following significant findings: patients with heart

failure without pulmonary hypertension were at significantly lower risk for mortality than those with pulmonary hypertension; and in patients with and without pulmonary hypertension, ongoing knowledge of PAP data resulted in a reduction in heart failure hospitalizations.

Left Atrial Pressure Monitors

An implantable system for the direct measurement of LAP has been developed[26,27] and is under ongoing investigation. The system consists of an implantable sensor lead coupled to a subcutaneous antenna coil, a patient advisory module, and remote clinician access via a secure computer-based data management system. Using a transvenous approach and transseptal crossing of the interatrial septum, the tip of the sensor system lead is oriented to the left atrium, providing

Table 1
Heart failure hospitalization rates at 6 months by baseline LVEF in the CHAMPION trial

Ejection Fraction	Randomization Group	6 Mo Rates of Hospitalization for Heart Failure	Incidence Rate Ratio (95% Confidence Interval) [P Value]
≥40%	Treatment group (N = 62)	0.18	0.54 (0.38–0.70) [P<.0001]
	Control group (N = 57)	0.33	
≥50%	Treatment group (N = 35)	0.18	0.50 (0.29–0.86) [P = .0129]
	Control group (N = 31)	0.35	
<40%	Treatment group (N = 208)	0.36	0.76 (0.61–0.91) [P = .0085]
	Control group (N = 222)	0.47	

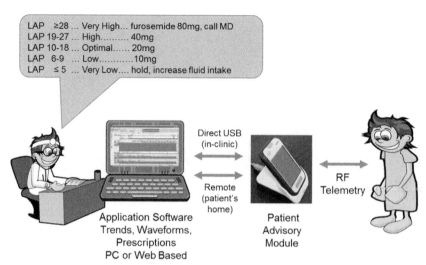

Fig. 4. Physician-directed, patient self-management of intracardiac pressure or PAP. Within physician-prescribed guidelines, patients with heart failure may one day manage their own intracardiac pressure or PAP like the approach shown. This approach is similar to how patients with diabetes use glucometers to self-manage their diabetes medications. The example shown uses LAP to monitor and manage heart failure.

measurement of LAP, temperature, and an intracardiac electrogram. The implant is powered and interrogated through the skin by wireless transmissions from the patient advisory module, and high-fidelity LAP waveforms are captured and stored in the patient advisory module.

Using the physician-directed, patient self-management approach depicted in **Fig. 4**, a prospective, observational, first-in-human study of this LAP monitoring system provided preliminary evidence of efficacy.[28] In this study, LAP monitoring improved hemodynamics, symptoms, and outcomes in NYHA class III and class IV patients with heart failure. Following a 3-month blinding period, LAP and individualized therapy instructions guided by these pressures were disclosed to the patient. The mean daily LAP decreased from 17.6 mm Hg in the first 3 months to 14.8 mm Hg ($P<.003$) during pressure-guided therapy. The frequency of readings greater than 25 mm Hg was reduced by 67% ($P<.001$). LVEF and NYHA class improved. Compared with the year before LAP monitor implantation and with the 3-month period of observation postimplantation, the annualized rate of heart failure hospitalization was significantly reduced following initiation of the physician-directed, patient self-management approach. These findings are being evaluated further in a large prospective randomized controlled outcomes study.

SUMMARY

An implantable PAP measurement system was recently approved for the management of NYHA class III patients with heart failure with a history of heart failure hospitalization in the past 12 months. Therapy guided by knowledge of PAP significantly reduces the risk of heart failure hospitalization and improves quality of life in systolic and diastolic patients with heart failure. This ushers in a new era of heart failure management based on information derived from implantable hemodynamic monitoring systems. Other implantable hemodynamic monitoring systems are under investigation, as is the approach of physician-directed, patient self-management based on direct measurement of intracardiac pressure or PAP.

REFERENCES

1. Go AS, Mozaffarian D, Roger VL, et al. Heart disease and stroke statistics: 2014 update. A report from the American Heart Association. Circulation 2014;129:e27–292.
2. Jencks SF, Williams MV, Coleman EA. Rehospitalizations among patients in the Medicare fee-for-service program. N Engl J Med 2009;360:1418–28.
3. Ross JS, Chen J, Lin Z, et al. Recent national trends in readmission rates after heart failure hospitalization. Circ Heart Fail 2010;3:97–103.
4. Kociol RD, Hammill BG, Fonarow GC, et al. Generalizability and longitudinal outcomes of a national heart failure clinical registry: comparison of Acute Decompensated Heart Failure National Registry (ADHERE) and non-ADHERE Medicare beneficiaries. Am Heart J 2010;160:885–92.
5. Moser DK, Yamokoski L, Sun JL, et al. Improvement in health-related quality of life after hospitalization

predicts event-free survival in patients with advanced heart failure. J Card Fail 2009;15:763–9.

6. Heidenreich PA. Forecasting the impact of heart failure in the United States: a policy statement from the American Heart Association. Circ Heart Fail 2013;6: 606–19.

7. Klersy C, De Silvestri A, Gabutti G, et al. A meta-analysis of remote monitoring of heart failure patients. J Am Coll Cardiol 2009;54:1683–94.

8. Inglis SC, Clark RA, McAlister FA, et al. Structured telephone support or telemonitoring programmes for patients with chronic heart failure. Cochrane Database Syst Rev 2010;(8):CD007228.

9. Chaudhry SI, Mattera JA, Curtis JP, et al. Telemonitoring in patients with heart failure. N Engl J Med 2010;363:2301–9.

10. Koehler F, Winkler S, Schieber M, et al. Impact of remote telemedical management on mortality and hospitalizations in ambulatory patients with chronic heart failure: the Telemedical Interventional Monitoring in Heart Failure study. Circulation 2011;123: 1873–80.

11. Lewin J, Ledwidge M, O'Loughlin C, et al. Clinical deterioration in established heart failure: what is the value of BNP and weight gain in aiding diagnosis? Eur J Heart Fail 2005;7:953–7.

12. Abraham WT, Compton S, Haas G, et al. Intrathoracic impedance vs daily weight monitoring for predicting worsening heart failure events: results of the Fluid Accumulation Status Trial (FAST). Congest Heart Fail 2011;17:51–5.

13. Yu CM, Wang L, Chau E, et al. Intrathoracic impedance monitoring in patients with heart failure: correlation with fluid status and feasibility of early warning preceding hospitalization. Circulation 2005;112:841–8.

14. Ypenburg C, Bax JJ, van der Wall EE, et al. Intrathoracic impedance monitoring to predict decompensated heart failure. Am J Cardiol 2007;99:554–7.

15. Adamson PB, Smith AL, Abraham WT, et al. Continuous autonomic assessment in patients with symptomatic heart failure: prognostic value of heart rate variability measured by an implanted cardiac resynchronization device. Circulation 2004;110:2389–94.

16. Whellan DJ, Ousdigian KT, Al-Khatib SM, et al. Combined heart failure device diagnostics identify patients at higher risk of subsequent heart failure hospitalizations: results from PARTNERS HF (Program to Access and Review Trending Information and Evaluate Correlation to Symptoms in Patients With Heart Failure) study. J Am Coll Cardiol 2010; 55:1803–10.

17. Reynolds DW, Bartelt N, Taepke R, et al. Measurement of pulmonary artery diastolic pressure from the right ventricle. J Am Coll Cardiol 1995;25: 1176–82.

18. Adamson PB, Magalski A, Braunschweig F, et al. Ongoing right ventricular hemodynamics in heart failure: clinical value of measurements derived from an implantable monitoring system. J Am Coll Cardiol 2003;41:565–71.

19. Bourge RC, Abraham WT, Adamson PB, et al. Randomized controlled trial of an implantable continuous hemodynamic monitor in patients with advanced heart failure: the COMPASS-HF study. J Am Coll Cardiol 2008;51:1073–9.

20. Stevenson LW, Zile M, Bennett TD, et al. Chronic ambulatory intracardiac pressures and future heart failure events. Circ Heart Fail 2010;3:580–7.

21. Adamson PB, Abraham WT, Aaron M, et al. CHAMPION trial rationale and design: the long-term safety and clinical efficacy of a wireless pulmonary artery pressure monitoring system. J Card Fail 2011;17: 3–10.

22. Abraham WT, Adamson PB, Bourge RC, et al. Wireless pulmonary artery haemodynamic monitoring in chronic heart failure: a randomised controlled trial. Lancet 2011;377:658–66.

23. Abraham WT, Adamson PB, Hasan A, et al. Safety and accuracy of a wireless pulmonary artery pressure monitoring system in patients with heart failure. Am Heart J 2011;161:558–66.

24. Adamson PB, Abraham WT, Bourge RC, et al. Wireless pulmonary artery pressure monitoring guides management to reduce decompensation in heart failure with preserved ejection fraction. Circ Heart Fail 2014;7:935–44.

25. Benza RL, Raina A, Abraham WT, et al. Pulmonary hypertension related to left heart disease: insight from a wireless implantable hemodynamic monitor. J Heart Lung Transpl 2014. [Epub ahead of print].

26. Ritzema J, Melton IC, Richards AM, et al. Direct left atrial pressure monitoring in ambulatory heart failure patients: initial experience with a new permanent implantable device. Circulation 2007;116:2952–9.

27. Troughton RW, Ritzema J, Eigler NL, et al. Direct left atrial pressure monitoring in severe heart failure: long-term sensor performance. J Cardiovasc Transl Res 2011;4:3–13.

28. Ritzema J, Troughton R, Melton I, et al. Physician-directed patient self-management of left atrial pressure in advanced chronic heart failure. Circulation 2010;121:1086–95.

Contemporary Drug-Eluting Stent Platforms
Design, Safety, and Clinical Efficacy

Ramon A. Partida, MD[a,b,c],
Robert W. Yeh, MD, MSc, MBA[c,d,e],*

KEYWORDS

- Drug-eluting stents • Percutaneous coronary intervention • Coronary stent
- Coronary artery disease • Drug-eluting stents: trends • Equipment design • Review

KEY POINTS

- Contemporary drug-eluting stent (DES) platforms have been developed to address high rates of restenosis seen with bare-metal stents and late adverse events seen with first-generation DES.
- Contemporary DES platforms incorporate significant advances in scaffold design, polymer compatibility, and antiproliferative drug delivery.
- DES use has become the standard of care in most clinical scenarios during percutaneous coronary intervention, including high-risk settings.

INTRODUCTION

Percutaneous coronary intervention (PCI) technology has advanced significantly since the first balloon angioplasty by Gruentzig in 1977 and eventually the first stent implantation in a patient by Sigwart and colleagues[1] 1 year later.

Initial efforts with balloon angioplasty were fraught with exceedingly high rates of restenosis, dissection, and abrupt vessel closure. These initial issues led to the development of the bare-metal stent (BMS) to scaffold vessels, leading to increased acute coronary artery luminal gain and maintenance of luminal integrity. Significant improvement in acute clinical outcomes was noted following the use of BMS, with a 20% to 30% decrease in clinical and angiographic restenosis.[2] However, vessel response to stent-mediated vascular injury leads to a significant amount of neointimal hyperplasia, vascular smooth muscle cell migration, and proliferation. This, in turn, leads to negative remodeling, restenosis, and late luminal loss, portending a high risk of need for reintervention.

The drug-eluting stent (DES) was developed to minimize the risk of in-stent restenosis. First-generation DESs have consistently been shown to decrease the risk of restenosis and need for reintervention compared with the BMS.[3] Despite proven clinical efficacy in the treatment of coronary disease, reports of adverse clinical outcomes,

This article originally appeared in Interventional Cardiology Clinics, Volume 5, Issue 3, July 2016.
Disclosures: R.A. Partida has no relevant disclosures. R.W. Yeh has served on scientific advisory boards and received consulting fees for Abbott Vascular and Boston Scientific.
[a] Division of Cardiology, Department of Medicine, Massachusetts General Hospital, 55 Fruit Street, GRB-800 Boston, MA 02114, USA; [b] Institute for Medical Engineering and Science, Massachusetts Institute of Technology, 77 Massachusetts Avenue, E25-438, Cambridge, MA 02139, USA; [c] Harvard Medical School, 25 Shattuck Street, Boston, MA 02115, USA; [d] Department of Medicine, Smith Center for Outcomes Research in Cardiology, CardioVascular Institute, Beth Israel Medical Center, 330 Brookline Avenue, Baker 4, Boston, MA 02215, USA; [e] Harvard Clinical Research Institute, Boston, MA, USA
* Corresponding author. Smith Center for Outcomes Research in Cardiology, CardioVascular Institute, Beth Israel Medical Center, 330 Brookline Avenue, Baker 4, Boston, MA 02215.
E-mail address: ryeh@bidmc.harvard.edu

mostly related to stent thrombosis (ST) and late restenosis, raised concerns regarding DES safety and limitation of these devices. Since the initial experience with first-generation DES, significant improvements have occurred with current DES platform technology, leading to increased safety and efficacy.[4–6] Additionally, although not the focus of this article, concurrent advances in adjunct pharmacotherapy and antiplatelet therapy have resulted in improved clinical outcomes. The sections that follow focus on the design improvements of the contemporary DES, as well as the clinical safety and efficacy of current stent platforms approved for use by the Federal Drug Administration (FDA).

COMPONENT DESIGN

DES platforms consist of 3 main components: (1) a stent metallic platform or scaffold, (2) a stent polymer coating that allows for controlled drug release, and (3) a released antiproliferative drug. **Fig. 1** shows a representative schematic the DES components.

Metallic Stent Scaffold

Current FDA-approved DES platforms are based on metallic scaffolds made of biologically inert metals with high radial strength. First-generation stents used stainless steel (SS) as the metal of choice. Recent research and development efforts have also included development of fully resorbable scaffold materials, which are currently undergoing preclinical and clinical investigation.

Although a breadth of research has focused on the advancement of polymer and antiproliferative drug components, significant improvement has also been achieved in the development of these metallic stent scaffolds. Generally, stent scaffolds are composed of 2 main components: hoops in series to provide radial strength on expansion, and connectors that join these hoops and provide longitudinal strength.[7,8] Early clinical experience, as well as insight obtained from preclinical and computational models, shed light on the role of stent geometry and strut size in deliverability; stent visibility; drug deposition; and, importantly, clinical outcomes and restenosis risk.

Initial efforts focused on optimizing stent design with existing alloys 316L-SS, such as the TAXUS Liberté stent platform (Boston Scientific, Natick, MA, USA). This allowed for reduced strut thickness of 100 to 140 μm with preserved radial strength. However, further improvement was limited by the material's moderate yield and limited compression

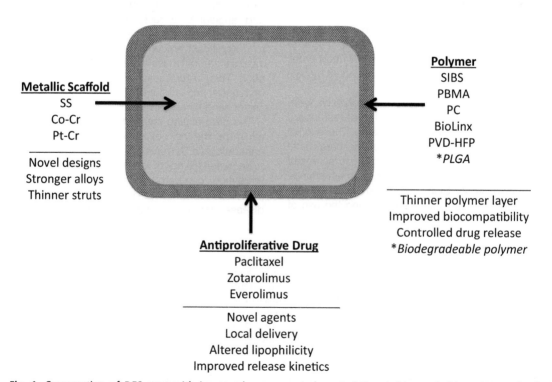

Metallic Scaffold
SS
Co-Cr
Pt-Cr
———————
Novel designs
Stronger alloys
Thinner struts

Polymer
SIBS
PBMA
PC
BioLinx
PVD-HFP
PLGA
———————
Thinner polymer layer
Improved biocompatibility
Controlled drug release
Biodegradeable polymer

Antiproliferative Drug
Paclitaxel
Zotarolimus
Everolimus
———————
Novel agents
Local delivery
Altered lipophilicity
Improved release kinetics

Fig. 1. Cross-section of DES strut with improved component characteristics. *, bioresorbable polymer; Co–Cr, cobalt–chromium; PBMA, poly(n-butyl methacrylate); PC, phosphorylcholine; PLGA, poly(lactic-co-glycolic acid); Pt–Cr, platinum–chromium; PVDF-HFP, copolymer of vinylidene fluoride and hexafluoropropylene; SIBS, poly(styrene-b-isobutylene-b-styrene); SS, stainless steel.

strength and visibility. Cobalt–chromium (Co–Cr) alloys used in the Vision (Abbott Vascular, Santa Clara, CA) and Driver (Medtronic, Minneapolis, MN) stent platforms have higher yield strength and modestly higher radiopacity compared with SS, and allowed for further reduction in strut thickness of 80 to 90 μm, albeit with higher elastic properties. Similarly, platinum–chromium (Pt–Cr) alloys (Promus Element and TAXUS Element stent platform) allowed for similar reduction in strut thickness and higher radiopacity given this alloy's higher yield strength.[9,10] All 3 of these alloys have been shown to be biocompatible and equivalent in in vivo preclinical models.[11] **Fig. 2** depicts the stent design and major characteristic of currently available scaffold platforms.

In summary, the development of scaffolds made with these alternative metallic alloys allowed for scaffolds with smaller strut profiles with similar stent radial strength and visibility under fluoroscopy. These developments have been shown to be associated with lesser degree of arterial damage during deployment, likely reducing a stimuli for restenosis.[9,12] This holds true independent of stent geometric design.[13] In addition, scaffolds with thinner struts and decreased number of hoop connectors allow for improved device flexibility, conformability to the blood vessel, and deliverability to the target lesion; as well as theoretic improved side branch access given decreased overall scaffold profile.[7,14] Some of these design parameters seem important, not only for procedural and acute technical

success, but as key drivers of drug delivery to local tissue. Stent conformability to the target vessel, stable scaffold geometric configuration, and polymer characteristics are some of the important determinants of the distribution of eluted drug.[6,15–17]

Stent Polymer Coating

Stent polymer coatings are applied to the metallic scaffold and act as drug carriers that allow for controlled local drug delivery. All except 1 of the currently FDA-approved platforms contain durable, synthetic polymer coatings that allow for predictable drug elution pharmacokinetics.

Concerns arising from reports of late ST, poor re-endothelialization, and potential hypersensitivity reactions with the use of first-generation DES platforms[18,19] led to the development of more highly biocompatible permanent polymers seen in contemporary platforms. These have been designed to induce minimal thrombogenicity at the stent surface, decrease vessel wall injury, allow for differential drug-release profiles, and lead to significant reduction in polymer layer thickness (by 40%–70%) thus decreasing the overall effective strut thickness (metal strut thickness plus polymer layer).[9] Of note, all of the currently approved DES platforms have circumferential polymer and drug elution along each strut.

More recent research has been aimed at platforms with biodegradable polymers that resorb after drug elution. The Synergy bioabsorbable

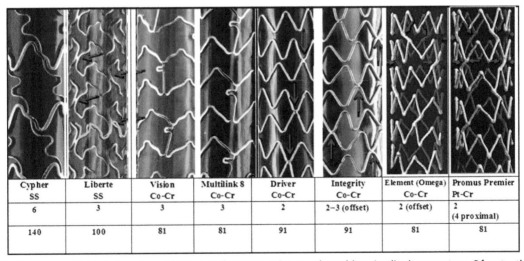

Cypher SS	Liberte SS	Vision Co-Cr	Multilink 8 Co-Cr	Driver Co-Cr	Integrity Co-Cr	Element (Omega) Co-Cr	Promus Premier Pt-Cr
6	3	3	3	2	2–3 (offset)	2 (offset)	2 (4 proximal)
140	100	81	81	91	91	81	81

Fig. 2. Stent scaffold design characteristics. Red arrows point to selected longitudinal connectors. Of note, the Promus Premier platform is identical to the Promus Element design except for the presence of 2 instead of 4 connectors in the proximal stent hoops. (*Adapted from* Ormiston JA, Webber B, Webster MW. Stent longitudinal integrity bench insights into a clinical problem. JACC Cardiovasc Interv 2011;4:1312; and Ormiston JA, Webber B, Ubod B, et al. Coronary stent durability and fracture: an independent bench comparison of six contemporary designs using a repetitive bend test. EuroIntervention 2015;12:1450.)

polymer (BP)-DES (Boston Scientific, Natick, MA, USA), consists of a Pt–Cr scaffold of 74 μm strut thickness, with a biodegradable poly(lactic-co-glycolic acid) (PLGA) polymer of 4 μm thickness on the abluminal surface. The polymer and drug are eluted over 4 months, after which only the metallic scaffold remains.[20] In October 2015, this platform was the first BP-DES to receive FDA approval for clinical use based on the results of the EVOLVE II trial; however, it is not yet in widespread clinical use.[20] Additional BP-DESs, such as the sirolimus-eluting Orsiro (Biotronik, Berlin, Germany), the biolimus-eluting Nobori (Terumo Corporation, Tokyo, Japan), and the novolimus-eluting DESyne BD (Elixir Medical, Sunnyvale, CA, USA), which have received the European Conformity (CE) mark but are not yet FDA approved, are outside the scope of this article.[3,21] Recent preclinical and early clinical research has focused on the use of polymer-free platforms with the use of microfabricated and nanofabricated reservoirs on the stent scaffold surface.[21]

Released Antiproliferative Drug

The eluted antiproliferative drugs are the third component of the DES platform. These are embedded in the stent polymer and are distributed into the vessel wall via diffusion in a manner dictated by local flow parameters and polymer characteristics. In this manner, the drug and polymer determine the characteristics of the vascular response and time course of vascular healing.[22]

Stent implantation induces local mechanical injury to the arterial wall and endothelium, forming a nidus for platelet activation, thrombus formation, and recruitment of monocytes, and ultimately leading to smooth muscle cell proliferation and neointimal hyperplasia.[9] Antiproliferative agents target this cellular response to reduce the rates of neointimal hyperplasia and restenosis. The main agents currently in clinical use include sirolimus analogues and paclitaxel.[3]

Paclitaxel binds to and acts as a microtubule-stabilizing agent preventing smooth muscle cell proliferation. Sirolimus and its analogues bind to the intracellular receptor of FKBP12 to inhibit the mammalian target of rapamycin, resulting in inhibition of vascular smooth muscle migration and proliferation. Additionally, it is a potent inhibitor of endothelial cell proliferation.[3,21,22] Zotarolimus is a more lipophilic analogue of sirolimus and was the first medication developed specifically for the treatment of in-stent restenosis. Everolimus is another sirolimus analogue with a shorter pharmacokinetic half-life.[3,21]

Recent preclinical research has also included the use of dual DESs that combine an antiproliferative agent with either an antithrombotic re-endothelialization promoter or a second antiproliferative agent.[21] Other novel antiproliferative agents have been developed, including novolimus (sirolimus metabolite developed for stent use), biolimus (a more hydrophilic analogue of sirolimus), and myolimus (a rapamycin derivative), which are currently being tested in early clinical trials.[9,23]

In summary, the combination of design improvements on metallic stent scaffolds, polymer technology, and antiproliferative drugs have allowed for newer generation DES platforms with improved scaffold mechanics, polymer biocompatibility, and drug-release kinetics for improved vascular endothelial healing, which have led to improved safety and clinical performance (see later discussion). Currently available DES platforms combine different scaffold designs, scaffold materials, polymers, and antiproliferative drugs, as summarized in **Table 1**.

COMMERCIALLY AVAILABLE, CONTEMPORARY, FIRST-GENERATION DRUG-ELUTING STENT PLATFORMS

This section provides an overview of DES platforms approved for use in the United States by the FDA, with a focus on their platform design characteristics and latest clinical safety and efficacy data.

The TAXUS Express and Cypher (Cordis, Miami Lakes, FL, USA) DES are examples of first-generation platforms that established the foundation for the development of newer-generation DES. The TAXUS paclitaxel-eluting stent (PES) consisted of a SS scaffold with a 132 μm strut plus 22 μm polymer thickness, whereas the Cypher sirolimus-eluting stent (SES) consisted of a SS scaffold of 140 μm strut thickness with a 13 μm polymer layer. These first-generation stents served as main comparators to contemporary DES in multiple clinical trials (see later discussion).

The TAXUS Liberté is a PES on a SS hybrid design scaffold with a strut thickness of 97 μm with a 16 μm thick layer of triblock polymer matrix of poly(styrene-b-isobutylene-b-styrene) and a paclitaxel concentration of 10 μg/mm2 with very slow drug-release kinetics, leading to less than 10% paclitaxel elution during the initial 28 days.[24] The TAXUS Element PES (ION stent) is a next-generation system with the same polymer and drug components on a Pt–Cr open cell design scaffold of 81 μm strut thickness (Element scaffold design) that was approved by the FDA in 2011.[26]

Table 1
Current drug-eluting stent platforms

Stent Name	Cypher (1st Generation)	TAXUS Express (1st Generation)	TAXUS Liberte	TAXUS Element (ION)	Endeavor	Resolute	Xience V Xpedition	Promus Element	Promus Premier	Synergy
Scaffold Alloy	SS	SS	SS	Pt–Cr	Co–Cr	Co–Cr	Co–Cr	Co–Cr	Pt–Cr	Pt–Cr
Drug (concentration, g/cm²)	Sirolimus (140)	Paclitaxel (100)	Paclitaxel (100)	Paclitaxel (100)	Zotarolimus (160)	Zotarolimus (160)	Everolimus (100)	Everolimus (100)	Everolimus (100)	Everolimus (100)
Release Kinetics	80% over 30 d	<10% over 10 d: 90% unreleased	<10% over 10 d: 90% unreleased	<10% over 10 d: 90% unreleased	95% over 14 d	80% over 60 d; 100% over 6 mo	80% over 30 d 100% over 6 mo	80% over 30 d; 100% over 6 mo	80% over 30 d; 100% over 6 mo	50% over 30 d; 80% over 2 mo
Scaffold Design	Cypher Select	Express	Liberte	Element	Driver	Driver	Multi-Link 8	Element	Promus Premier	Element
Strut Thickness (μm)	140	132	97	81	91	91	81	81	81	74
Polymer Thickness (μm)	13	22	16	15	6	6	8	8	8	4 (Abluminal)
Polymer	PEVA/PBMA	SIBS	SIBS	SIBS	PC	BioLinx	PBMA, PVDF-HFP	PBMA, PVDF-HFP	PBMA, PVDF-HFP	Bioabsorbable PLGA
Manufacturer	Cordis	Boston Scientific	Boston Scientific	Boston Scientific	Medtronic	Medtronic	Abbott Vascular	Boston Scientific	Boston Scientific	Boston Scientific
FDA Approval	2003 (no longer available)	2004 (no longer available)	2004	2011	2008	2012	2008	2008	2013	2015

Key component characteristics of current commercially available DES platforms in the United States with select first-generation DES (no longer available).
Abbreviations: HFP, hexafluoropropylene; PBMA, poly(n-butyl methacrylate); PC, phosphorylcholine; PEVA, polyethylene-co-vinyl acetate; PLGA, poly(lactic-co-glycolic acid); PVDF, polyvinylidene fluoride; SIBS, poly(styrene-b-isobutylene-b-styrene).
Data from Refs.[3,9,14,24,25]

The Endeavor (Medtronic, Minneapolis, MN, USA) platform is a zotarolimus-eluting stents (ZES) consisting of a Co–Cr open cell scaffold of 91 μm strut thickness and a 6 μm polymer layer thickness. It contains a zotarolimus concentration of 10 μg/mm stent length (or 160 g/cm^2) and a highly biocompatible hydrophilic phosphorylcholine polymer that results in very rapid drug-elution profile, with greater than 95% eluted in the initial 14 days postimplantation.[14,25]

The Resolute Integrity ZES (Medtronic, Minneapolis, MN, USA) has the same metallic scaffold and drug concentration as the Endeavor ZES (E-ZES) but contains a BioLinx polymer that is highly biocompatible and provides slower release kinetics with 85% of drug eluted over 2 months and complete elution by 6 months.[14,25]

The Xience Alpine (Xpeditition or Xience Prime) (Abbott Vascular, Santa Clara, CA, USA) is a Co–Cr everolimus-eluting stent (EES) of 81 μm strut and 8 μm polymer thickness on a multilink stent open cell platform and Promus DES built on a Vision stent platform. It contains 100 g/cm^2 everolimus concentration on an acrylic and fluorinated polymer that allows for 80% of the drug to be eluted in the first 2 months postimplantation and completely by 6 months.[3,14]

The Promus Premier (Boston Scientific, Natick, MA, USA) is a Pt–Cr EES 81 μm strut thickness and 8 μm polymer thickness on an Element open cell stent platform. The polymer, drug concentration and elution characteristics are otherwise the same as the Xience Alpine Co–Cr EES.[14,25]

Table 1 shows a summary of the current commercially available stents in the United States (stent name, scaffold material, scaffold design, strut thickness, polymer, drug concentration, drug elution kinetics, FDA-approval year, and manufacturer).[3,9,14,24,25]

DEVICE-RELATED SAFETY OUTCOMES: INSIGHTS FROM MECHANICAL AND DEVICE INTEGRITY AND FAILURE
Stent Fracture

The safety of contemporary DES platforms can be evaluated from 2 distinct perspectives: (1) a device-centric model, centered on the risk of adverse events secondary to type of drug released or to mechanical device failure as determined by stent strut fracture and stent longitudinal deformation; and (2) a clinical standpoint, centered on the risk of ST and risk for target lesion revascularization (TLR).

Certain device specific characteristics have been associated with adverse clinical events. For example, certain risk factors have been recognized

to increase the risk of strut fracture, which in turn has been shown to be related to higher rates of clinically evident restenosis, ST, aneurysm formation, myocardial infarction (MI), and TLR.[27–30] Some of the recognized risk factors for stent fracture include lesion complexity (eg, length, degree of calcification, vessel tortuosity, and angulation), deployment characteristic (overlapping stents, higher inflation pressure), and anatomic location (hinge points, right coronary artery, or ostial implantation).[28,30–32] Current research is ongoing in further understanding the causes, mechanisms, and underlying microenvironment stresses and strains driving this phenomenon and associated complications.[32]

Stent fracture is an uncommon complication, with a historical incidence ranging between 0.9% and 8.4%, with a 4.0% incidence on recent meta-analysis of over 5000 subjects.[31] Importantly, however, first-generation DES platforms with a SS closed-cell stent design and sirolimus elution were included and represented approximately 90% of the reported cases, while the remaining 10% were evenly distributed among all the contemporary platforms.[29] A separate registry analysis of over 9000 subjects reported a strut fracture incidence rate of 1.25% in contemporary platforms.[33] Improvement in stent design, with reduction of the number of connectors between rings from 6 S-connectors (first-generation DES, leading to decreased flexibility, stiffer stent frame) to 2 to 3 connectors in contemporary DES designs, have been largely responsible for these observations of decreased fracture despite decreasing strut thickness.

Longitudinal Deformation

Longitudinal deformation has been discussed as another potential mechanical complication of novel stent platforms, particularly given the shift toward open cell designs to allow for improved trackability while maintaining radial strength. These designs have decreased number of interconnectors between the stent rings and have been a perceived higher risk of longitudinal stent deformation or pseudofracture, which appears most commonly in the Element platform design with its distinct offset peak-to-peak interconnected ring design.[34] Although clinical outcomes with Pt–Cr EES Promus Element are similar to other second-generation DESs, bench studies suggest the Promus Element stent design has decreased longitudinal strength, making it potentially vulnerable to longitudinal shortening.[7]

Limited data are available regarding the incidence and associated clinical outcomes from longitudinal stent deformation but, in limited series, it occurs in 0.1% to 1.0% of contemporary DES platforms. It seems to be related to stent design characteristics, with a higher incidence for the offset peak-to-peak design (Promus Element platform) observed both clinically in limited, retrospective analyses[35] and in in vitro engineering longitudinal compression models.[7,36] Of note and as expected, longitudinal deformation was rarely observed with the stiffer early-generation DES platforms. Despite reports of increased risk of longitudinal deformation with novel thin-strut stents and potential association to ST[35] it seems to be a rare occurrence[37] that is mostly related to attempts to pass equipment through secondary devices during PCI.[34]

Pathologic Correlates of Stent Fracture

Pathologic and autopsy studies have shed additional light into the clinical significance of this problem. Although historical incidence was reported at 1% to 2%, autopsy studies have reported a higher incidence. However, only the most severe types of stent fractures causing gaps in stented segments were associated with adverse histologic findings on pathologic studies.[30] Contemporary Co–Cr EES platforms also seem to have decreased risk of strut fracture despite the thinner strut profiles compared with PES or SES and improved strut coverage with less evidence of inflammation, fibrin deposition, and late and very late ST (VLST). Despite these pathologic findings, fracture-related restenosis or thrombosis was comparable.[38]

Patient-Related Safety Outcomes: Insights from Clinical Experience

From a clinical perspective, and as previously discussed, first-generation DES platforms markedly decreased the risk of restenosis and have led to improved clinical outcomes. The safety of first-generation and contemporary DES platforms has centered mostly on the risk of ST. It represents a rare but potentially serious complication with a high morbidity and mortality.[39,40] First-generation DES platforms were found to have similar rates of early (0–30 days) and late (31–360 days) ST compared with the BMS.[5,41] However, safety concerns arose with reports of significantly increased, and persistent, annual risk of VLST of approximately 0.5% for up to 5 years postimplantation compared with BMS,[5,42,43] albeit with a lower restenosis and subsequent MI risk.[44]

Pathologic studies shed insight these complications because late ST and VLST seem to have distinct mechanisms between SES and PES platforms. Interestingly, SES specimens showed evidence of a hypersensitivity reaction with diffuse extensive inflammation, whereas PES specimens showed late stent malapposition with excessive fibrin deposition.[45]

Second-generation DES, with their improvements in scaffold design, polymer biocompatibility, and antiproliferative drug content, concentration, and elution kinetics, have significantly decreased this risk by addressing these failure mechanisms: pathologic studies of contemporary EES platforms have been shown to result in improved strut coverage and endothelialization, resulting in a decreased inflammatory response, less fibrin deposition, and decreased evidence of late and VLST compared with first-generation SES and PES in human autopsy analysis.[38]

A large network meta-analysis of 52,158 subjects enrolled in 51 trials with follow-up of at least 3 years, compared the long-term safety of DES to BMS up to a mean of 3.8 years, and found improved efficacy and safety profile of DES with lower rates of definite ST and target vessel revascularization (TVR), with improved efficacy of Co–Cr EES compared with earlier generation DES platforms.[46] Of note, although the EXAMINATION (A Clinical Evaluation of Everolimus Eluting Coronary Stents in the Treatment of Patients With ST-segment Elevation Myocardial Infarction) trial did not demonstrate superiority of Co–Cr EES to BMS with respect to subject-oriented endpoints in the ST-segment elevation MI (STEMI) population at 1-year follow-up, 5-year follow-up data demonstrated lower rates of these endpoints, including all-cause mortality. Importantly, TLR and ST rates were consistently lower with DES.[47,48]

In addition to meta-analyses, data from a recent large, randomized study of dual antiplatelet therapy duration has shed additional light into the safety of contemporary DES platforms. A prospective, propensity-matched analysis of subjects enrolled in the dual antiplatelet therapy (DAPT) study comparing 12 and 30 months of dual antiplatelet in 10,026 subjects (8308 with DES vs 1718 with BMS) showed a lower risk of ST with DES compared with BMS (1.7% vs 2.6%, $P = .01$).[49]

CLINICAL EFFICACY OF SPECIFIC STENT PLATFORMS
Paclitaxel-Eluting Stents

The first-generation TAXUS Express SS-PES has been found to have increasing rates of VLST compared with BMS, with reduced risk of restenosis balancing out overall clinical risk of death and MI.[42] The TAXUS Element (ION stent) represents the latest-generation Pt–Cr PES platform, which was tested against the TAXUS Express platform

(SS-PES) and shown to be noninferior in the randomized PERSEUS-WH (A Prospective Evaluation in a Randomized Trial of the Safety and Efficacy of the Use of the TAXUS Element Paclitaxel-Eluting Coronary Stent System for the Treatment of De Novo Coronary Artery Lesions) clinical trial, showing no differences in angiographic target lesion failure (TLF) or clinical outcomes out to 5 years.[50] In addition, PERSEUS-SV (A Prospective Evaluation in a Non-Randomized Trial of the Safety and Efficacy of the Use of the TAXUS Element Paclitaxel-Eluting Coronary Stent System for the Treatment of De Novo Coronary Artery Lesions in Small Vessels) was a second arm of the study comparing the TAXUS Element PES against BMS with the use of historical controls from the TAXUS IV and V trials. It showed significantly lower TLR (27.2% BMS vs 14.9% Pt–Cr PES; $P = .049$) and similar low rates of ST between them (0.5%–1.0%).[50]

Newer DES platforms, however, have been found to be superior to PES platforms in multiple large clinical studies and meta-analyses, with significantly lower risks of VLST and improved event-free survival on long-term follow-up.[5,51,52] In the SPIRIT III trial (A Clinical Evaluation of the Investigational Device XIENCE V Everolimus Eluting Coronary Stent System (EECSS) in the Treatment of Subjects With de Novo Native Coronary Artery Lesions) of 1002 subjects randomized 2 to 1 to Co–Cr EES versus SS-PES, EES was found to be superior in both angiographic endpoint of in-segment late loss at 8 months, as well as composite clinical endpoint of major adverse cardiac events (MACEs) due to lower rates of MI and TLR. These results were confirmed on final 5-year follow-up.[53,54] Similarly, the SPIRIT IV trial randomized 3687 subjects to EES or PES, and showed lower rates of the primary endpoint of TLF at 1 year with EES (relative risk [RR] 0.62; CI 0.46–0.82) compared with PES.[55] Furthermore, these results are consistent with the findings from a recent meta-analyses of the final results from the SPIRIT clinical trials program showing reduced rates of all-cause mortality, MI, ischemia-drive TLR, ST, and TLF with EES.[56] Recently, the Taxus Element versus Xience Prime in a Diabetic Population (TUXEDO)-India trial randomized the latest Pt–Cr PES platform to its contemporary Co–Cr EES platform in 1830 diabetic subjects, and PES failed to show noninferiority compared with EES in the study's primary endpoint of target vessel failure (TVF) (RR 1.89, CI 1.20–2.99, $P = .38$ for noninferiority). It showed higher rates of MI, ST, TVF, and TVL at 1-year follow-up with PES.[57]

Zotarolimus-Eluting Stents

The E-ZES platform was initially compared with its BMS scaffold base (Driver stent) and found to have lower rates of TLR in angiographic follow-up at 1 year (35.0% BMS vs 13.2% ZES, $P<.0001$) (ENDEAVOR II trial). These findings launched the ENDEAVOR clinical program, and ultimately the device's FDA approval in 2008 based on the results from the ENDEAVOR IV trial. This trial randomized subjects with de novo coronary lesions to treatment with E-ZES versus first-generation PES implantation and showed similar clinical safety and efficacy (noninferiority) in TLF despite a higher nonsignificant trend toward increased in-segment restenosis with ZES.[58] There were no differences in cardiac death, MI, TVR, or ST at 1-year follow-up. Importantly, at 5 year follow-up, there were no differences in rates of TLR (ZES 7.7% vs PES 8.6%, $P = .70$), TVF (17.2% vs 21.1%, $P = .061$); however, the rate of cardiac death or MI was lower with ZES (6.4% vs 9.1%, $P = .048$), driven by a lower rate of target vessel MI with ZES (2.6% vs 6.0%, $P = .002$). From a safety perspective, there was no difference in overall ST rates (ZES 1.3% vs PES 2%, $P = .42$); however, the rates of VLST (0.4% vs 1.8%, $P = .012$) and late MI events (1.3% vs 3.5%, $P = .008$) were significantly decreased with the use of ZES.[59]

The E-ZES platform was compared in a randomized trial to other early-generation DES with initial mixed results. E-ZES failed to meet its primary angiographic endpoint in the ENDEAVOR III trial owing to greater angiographic late loss compared with SES platforms, despite similar clinical endpoints at up to 5-year follow-up.[60] The larger ENDEAVOR IV trial eventually led to its FDA approval, whereas E-ZES was found to be noninferior to PES in a larger randomized trial with clinically oriented endpoints, although a trend toward VLST and late MI was observed in secondary analyses.[59] Subsequent trials had mixed results. The large 2333 subject SORT OUT III (Randomized Clinical Comparison of the Endeavor and the Cypher Coronary Stents in Non-selected Angina Pectoris Patients) trial in an unrestricted subject population showing higher rates of cardiac death, MI, and TVR (6% vs 3%, $P = .0002$). There were also higher rates of ST, MI, and TLR at 18 months, which leveled off and equalized owing to a higher rate of VLST with SES platforms at 3 year follow-up.[61] Further trials, however, showed higher degrees of angiographic restenosis but no increased rates of clinical events (death, MI, and ST) with E-ZES compared with SES[62] and when compared against either SES or PES.[63] In fact, a meta-analysis of these trials including 2132 subjects point to a favorable safety profile of the E-ZES compared with BMS, with very low rates of VSLT, MI, and cardiac death at 5 years; and with lower rates of TLR with ZES.[64] In the final 5-year follow-up of the E-ZES clinical trial program, E-ZES was found to have higher TLR at 1 year compared with first-generation DES; however, between 1 and 5 years, E-ZES was found to have significantly lower rates of TLR, cardiac death, MI, and ST.[65,66] Similarly, the PROTECT (Patient Related OuTcomes With Endeavor Versus Cypher Stenting Trial) trial showed a significantly lower risk of overall ST with ZES compared with SES (ZES 1.6% vs PES 2.6%, $P = .003$), with an improved safety profile and lower rates of VLST with E-ZES compared with SES at 4-year follow-up.[67]

The Resolute ZES, with its next-generation polymer allowing for slower zotarolimus-release kinetics, was initially evaluated in the pivotal, single-arm RESOLUTE (A Randomized Comparison of a Zotarolimus-Eluting Stent With an Everolimus-Eluting Stent for Percutaneous Coronary Intervention) trial, which showed angiographic restenosis rates of 2.1% at 9 months and 2-year TLR of 1.4% with no evidence of late ST.[68,69] This platform was subsequently evaluated against its contemporary Co–Cr EES platform (Xience V) in the RESOLUTE All-Comers trial of approximately 2300 subjects, showing similar 1-year rates of TLF (ZES 8.2% vs EES 8.3%, noninferiority $P = <0.001$), TLR (3.4% vs 3.9% $P = .50$), and ST (0.7% vs 1.6%, $P = .05$).[70] At 5-year follow-up, the rates of TLF, TLR, cardiac death, and MI were similar, as were rates of ST (2.8% vs 1.8%, $P = .12$).[71]

Most recently, the TWENTE (The Real-World Endeavor Resolute Versus XIENCE V Drug-Eluting Stent Study in Twente) trial randomized almost 1400 subjects from an unselected population with complex lesions (excluding high-risk lesions; eg, STEMI) to Resolute ZES and Xience V Co–Cr EES and showed similar rates of TVF (ZES 8.2% vs EES 8.1%, p noninferiority $= 0.001$), with similarly low ST rates (ZES 0.9% vs EES 1.2%, $P = .59$).[72]

In summary, these results and 2 recent studies comparing the Resolute ZES to newest generation Pt–Cr EES (see later discussion), show the Resolute ZES platform seems to have similar clinical efficacy and safety compared with contemporary EES platforms.

Everolimus-Eluting Stents

EES has been shown to be superior to BMS in the pivotal SPIRIT First trial, which compared Xience V Co–Cr EES with its identical Co–Cr BMS platform (Vision BMS), and showed markedly reduced rates of angiographic restenosis at 6 and 12 months.[73] It has also been shown to have a lower risk of ST compared with BMS in large meta-analyses.[74,75]

Compared with first-generation PES, the Co–Cr EES has consistently been shown to improve efficacy and safety. The pivotal SPIRIT III and SPIRIT IV trials compared the Co–Cr EES to PES and both showed decreased TLF (composite of cardiac death, MI, or TLR) at 1 year (3.9% vs 6.6%, $P = .0008$), with lower rates of ST (0.3% vs 1.1%, $P = .003$). Importantly, at 3 years, there seemed to be a decreased risk of mortality in the EES treatment arm, a finding that was confirmed at final 5-year follow-up with lower all-cause mortality (5.9% vs 10.1%, $P = .02$) and MACE (13.2% vs 20.7%, $P = .007$) with EES, despite lower but nonsignificant differences in ST, TLR, and MI.[54,55] This finding, however, has not been consistently reproduced. Another large trial (COMPARE [A Randomized Controlled Trial of Everolimus-eluting Stents and Paclitaxel-eluting Stents for Coronary Revascularization in Daily Practice]) showed improved efficacy and safety of EES compared with PES, driven instead by decreased rates of MI, TVR, and ST, without significant differences in mortality at 5-year follow-up. In this study, the rates of ST, MI, and TVR seemed to separate during the first 3 years, and then continued parallel thereafter.[76]

Randomized trials comparing Co–Cr EES with SES on the other hand, have not shown significant differences in clinical efficacy outcomes between the 2 platforms, with similar rates of TLR, MI, and death.[77–79] Differences have been observed, however, with lower rates of definite ST in EES compared with SES (0.2% vs 1.4%; HR 0.15, 95% CI 0.04–0.50) at 3-year follow-up in the SORT OUT IV trial of 2774 unselected subjects randomized to EES versus SES. As expected, this difference was driven mostly by a significant reduction in VLST with EES (0.1% vs 0.8%, HR 0.09, 95% CI 0.01–0.70).[80]

A large meta-analysis pooling more than 17,101 subjects from randomized control trials of EES versus PES or SES showed decreased rates of ST (RR 0.55, 95% CI 0.38–0.78), TVR (RR 0.77, 95% CI 0.64–0.92), and MI (RR 0.78, 95% CI 0.64–0.96) at a mean follow-up of almost 2 years.[81]

In summary, Co–Cr EES seems to have improved efficacy and safety compared with BMS and first-generation DES, driven by lower rates of ST and VLST. Although differences in clinical efficacy outcomes have generally not been observed in trials comparing EES to SES platforms, a large meta-analysis pooling over 17,000 subjects from studies of EES versus all non-EES platforms (PES, SES, or ZES), showed that EES was associated with significantly lower rates ST, MI, and TVR, albeit with no differences in cardiac mortality.

The Pt–Cr EES platform (Promus Element) has been shown to be noninferior to its Co–Cr EES analogue in its pivotal PLATINUM (A Prospective, Randomized, Multicenter Trial to Assess an Everolimus-Eluting Coronary Stent System (PROMUS Element) for the Treatment of up to Two De Novo Coronary Artery Lesions) trial randomizing 1530 subjects to Co–Cr EES or Pt–Cr EES at up to 3-year follow-up.[82,83]

The DUTCH PEERS (DUrable Polymer-based STent CHallenge of Promus Element Versus ReSolute Integrity in an All Comers Population) clinical trial compared the Resolute-ZES with Pt–Cr EES in a randomized, noninferiority trial enrolling 1811 subjects. It showed no significant difference in the primary combined endpoint of cardiac death, target vessel MI, and TLR at 12 months (ZES 6% vs EES 5%, noninferiority P <0.006), or in the rates of ST (ZES 0.7% vs 0.3% EES, P = .34). Interestingly, there were higher rates of longitudinal stent deformation with Pt–Cr EES (1.0%) than with Co–Cr ZES (0.0%, P = .002).[84]

Most recently, the Harmonizing Optimal Strategy for Treatment of Coronary Artery Stenosis-Safety and Effectiveness of Drug-Eluting Stents and Anti-Platelet Regimen (HOST-ASSURE) trial randomized 3755 subjects to Pt–Cr EES or Resolute Co–Cr ZES and showed no significant difference in TLF or clinical outcomes between the 2 groups (2.9% vs 2.9%). In contrast with prior studies, however, no differences were observed in rates of longitudinal stent deformation (Pt–Cr EES 0.2% vs Co–Cr ZES 0.0%), a concern owing to the scaffold design with thin struts and offset connectors leading to less longitudinal strength when tested in vitro (see previous discussion).[85]

Table 2 shows a selected list of randomized trials of contemporary DES platforms.

CLINICAL SAFETY AND EFFICACY IN SELECTED PATIENT POPULATIONS

The safety of contemporary DES platforms has increasingly been evaluated within specific populations of interest, including high-risk subsets such as acute MI, chronic kidney disease (CKD), and diabetes. Importantly, some of these high-risk populations are often excluded from many of the pivotal randomized trials.

Acute Myocardial Infarction

Stent implantation during acute coronary syndromes and MI remains a common clinical scenario for PCI, yet these patients were frequently excluded from many of the pivotal trials. It is associated with poorer outcomes. Initial results from first-generation DES raised concerns given significantly higher rates (RR 2.1 after 1 year) of VLST in this setting.[86] The dynamic environment during an acute coronary syndrome can lead to later stent malapposition due to thrombus, as well as potential delayed arterial healing from drug elution next to ruptured plaques.[43,87]

Computational and preclinical models shed additional mechanistic insight into potential causes for late failure with the use of DES because a thrombus present at the time of stent implantation during an acute MI modulates arterial drug distribution[88] and causes fluctuations in drug delivery.[89] Furthermore, similar models have shown that stent design (eg, thicker struts) and deployment are major drivers of thrombogenicity and appropriate polymer use reduces such risk, even in the setting of malapposition.[17]

Despite these concerns, contemporary DES platforms have been found to be safe and effective in this clinical setting. The EXAMINATION trial randomized 1498 subjects presenting with STEMI to treatment with Co–Cr EES (Xience V) versus BMS, and showed similar rates of combined subject-oriented endpoints of MI, all-cause death and revascularization, although rates of TLR were lower (EES 2.1% vs 5.0%, P = .003), as were rates of definite ST (0.5% vs 1.9%, P = .019).[48] Interestingly, at 5-year follow-up, subject-oriented clinical outcomes were significantly lower in the EES group (21%) compared with the BMS group (26%), driven mainly by reduced rate of all-cause mortality (EES 9% vs BMS 12%, P = .047).[47] Subsequent smaller studies have shown similar efficacy of EES compared with SES, albeit with lower rates of ST with EES platforms.[90,91]

Similarly, a network meta-analysis of 22 trials and 12,435 subjects with STEMI undergoing PCI with BMS, first-generation and second-generation DES (Pt–Cr EES excluded), confirmed an increasingly favorable safety and efficacy profile for DES, particularly with respect to Co–Cr EES platforms.[92] The exception in this clinical setting seemed to be the ZES platforms, which were found to have a significantly higher rate of TVR in this, as well as other separate analyses.[92,93]

Chronic Kidney Disease

Patients with CKD make up an increasingly large percentage, with over 40% in 1 retrospective

Table 2
Key selected trials of contemporary drug-eluting stents

Trial Name	Type of Study	Stents	Number of Subjects	Longest Follow-up (Years)	Primary Outcome	Key Exclusions	Key Results
SPIRIT III[55]	Multicenter, superiority RCT	PES vs Co-Cr EES (Xience)	1002	5	In-segment late loss at 9 mo	NSTEMI, STEMI	EES superior to PES angiographically Reduced MACE at 1, 5 y
SPIRIT IV[54]	Multicenter, superiority RCT	PES vs Co-Cr EES (Xience)	3687	5	TLF at 1 y	NSTEMI, STEMI	Lower all-cause mortality (5.9% vs 10.1%, $P = .02$) and MACE (13.2% vs 20.7%, $P = .007$) with EES
ENDEAVOR IV[59]	Multicenter, noninferiority	E-ZES vs PES	1548	—	TVF at 9 mo	NSTEMI, STEMI	E-ZES noninferior to PES Trend for increased VLST and late MI in secondary analyses
PROTECT[67]	—	E-ZES vs SES	8709	4	—	None	Lower risk of VLST and overall ST
RESOLUTE All-Comers[71]	Multicenter, noninferiority	Resolute ZES vs Co-Cr EES (Xience V)	2292	5	TLF	None	ZES noninferior to EES with similar rates of TLF, TLR, cardiac death and MI, and ST
COMPARE[76]	Single-center, superiority	Co-Cr EES vs ss-PES	1800	5	Death, MI, TVR at 1 y	None	EES with decreased rates of MI, TVR, ST without significant differences in mortality
SORT OUT IV[80]	RCT	Co-Cr EES vs SES	2774	3	CV death, MI, definite ST, TVR at 9 mo	None	EES with lower rates of definite ST (EES 0.2% vs SES 1.4%, HR: 0.15), and VLST (0.1% vs 0.8%, HR 0.09)
HOST-ASSURE[85]	Noninferiority, RCT	ZES vs Pt-Cr EES	3755	1	TLF at 1 y	None	No difference in TLF, clinical outcomes or rates of LSD
DUTCH PEERS[84]	RCT, noninferiority	Resolute ZES vs Pt-Cr EES	1811	1	Combined CV death, target vessel MI and TLR at 1 y	None	ZES noninferior to Pt-Cr EES Higher rates of LSD with Pt-Cr EES than Co-Cr ZES (1.0% vs 0.0%, $P = .002$)
TWENTE[72]	RCT, single-center, noninferiority	R-ZES vs Co-Cr EES (Xience-V)	1391	1	TVF	STEMI	ZES noninferior to EES Similar rates of TVF and ST
PLATINUM[83]	Multi-center, noninferiority RCT	Co-EES vs Pt-Cr EES	1530	3	TLF at 1 y	AMI	Pt-Cr EES noninferior to Co-Cr EES
PERSEUS-WH[50]	Multicenter, noninferiority RCT	Pt-Cr PES vs SS-PES	1264	5	TLF at 1 y	AMI	Similar rates of TLF (12.9% SS-PES vs 12.1% Pt-Cr PES, $P = .66$)
PERSEUS-SV[50]	Prospective multicenter, single-arm comparison	Pt-Cr PES vs BMS	224	5	Late lumen loss at 9 mo	AMI	Lower MACE and TLF with Pt-Cr PES driven by TLR

Selected key trials of contemporary DES highlighting key findings.
Abbreviations: HR, hazard ratio; LSD, longitudinal stent deformation; NSTEMI, non-STEMI; RCT, randomized clinical trial.
Data from Refs.[50,54,55,59,67,71,72,76,80,83–85]

series, of subjects undergoing PCI and DES implantation. Despite this, a scarcity of evidence exists to support its use.

Results from first-generation DES have failed to show improved efficacy compared with BMS in patients with mild to moderate CKD at up to 6-year follow-up and it has been suggested that the benefit of DES versus BMS in this population is attenuated by the altered vascular milieu.[94–96] It remains unclear whether contemporary DES use is associated with lower risk of restenosis or need for repeat revascularization compared with BMS[95] because there does not seem to be a significant difference in outcomes from DES versus BMS. As expected, a trend toward worse outcomes with PCI has been observed in the CKD population compared with patients with normal renal function.[94] Reassuringly, despite this decrease in clinical efficacy over BMS, DES use in this population has been proven to be as safe based on large retrospective propensity-matched cohort studies and registry analyses.[94–97]

Diabetes Mellitus

Diabetic patients also represent a high-risk population with historically high rates of restenosis and need for repeat revascularization. In diabetics, DES platforms have been found to have a similar safety profile to BMS if dual antiplatelet therapy is used for at least 6 months.[98] Similarly, they have been consistently been shown to have significantly lower rates of restenosis compared with BMS. A mixed-treatment comparison meta-analysis of 42 trials with 22,844 subject-years of follow-up concluded that all DES platforms were as safe as BMS (including rates of VLST) and had a significant reduction in rates of TVR (RR 37%–69%) compared with BMS.[99] Given the cumulative data, DES platforms are preferred to BMS for use in diabetic patients, although the specific DES platform of choice remains unclear. The Resolute ZES was the first to be approved by the FDA specifically for use in diabetic patients in 2012.[100] In 2015, the Promus Premier Pt–Cr EES also received FDA approval for use in patients with medically treated diabetes based on the results of the PROMUS Element Plus US Post Approval Study.

SUMMARY

DESs were developed in efforts to minimize the risk of in-stent restenosis seen with BMS. The initial concerns for high risk of late adverse events seen with first-generation DESs have significantly decreased with the use of contemporary platforms, owing to advances in scaffold design, novel

metallic alloys leading to thinner struts, polymer biocompatibility, and antiproliferative drug development and delivery. Several studies, including randomized controlled trials and meta-analyses, have consistently shown the efficacy and safety of contemporary DES platforms in both short-term and long-term follow-up. Given their proven efficacy and safety profile, the use of contemporary DESs has become standard in most clinical scenarios, including high-risk settings such as acute MI and diabetic population.

REFERENCES

1. Sigwart U, Puel J, Mirkovitch V, et al. Intravascular stents to prevent occlusion and restenosis after transluminal angioplasty. N Engl J Med 1987;316: 701–6.
2. Serruys PW, de Jaegere P, Kiemeneij F, et al. A comparison of balloon-expandable-stent implantation with balloon angioplasty in patients with coronary artery disease. Benestent Study Group. N Engl J Med 1994;331:489–95.
3. Stefanini GG, Holmes DR Jr. Drug-eluting coronary-artery stents. N Engl J Med 2013;368:254–65.
4. Cassese S, Piccolo R, Galasso G, et al. Twelve-month clinical outcomes of everolimus-eluting stent as compared to paclitaxel- and sirolimus-eluting stent in patients undergoing percutaneous coronary interventions. A meta-analysis of randomized clinical trials. Int J Cardiol 2011;150:84–9.
5. Raber L, Magro M, Stefanini GG, et al. Very late coronary stent thrombosis of a newer-generation everolimus-eluting stent compared with early-generation drug-eluting stents: a prospective cohort study. Circulation 2012;125:1110–21.
6. Garg S, Bourantas C, Serruys PW. New concepts in the design of drug-eluting coronary stents. Nat Rev Cardiol 2013;10:248–60.
7. Ormiston JA, Webber B, Webster MW. Stent longitudinal integrity bench insights into a clinical problem. JACC Cardiovasc Interv 2011;4:1310–7.
8. Ormiston JA, Webber B, Ubod B, et al. Stent longitudinal strength assessed using point compression: insights from a second-generation, clinically related bench test. Circ Cardiovasc Interv 2014;7: 62–9.
9. Martin DM, Boyle FJ. Drug-eluting stents for coronary artery disease: a review. Med Eng Phys 2011;33:148–63.
10. Sun D, Zheng Y, Yin T, et al. Coronary drug-eluting stents: from design optimization to newer strategies. J Biomed Mater Res A 2014;102:1625–40.
11. Menown IB, Noad R, Garcia EJ, et al. The platinum chromium element stent platform: from alloy, to design, to clinical practice. Adv Ther 2010;27: 129–41.

12. Kastrati A, Mehilli J, Dirschinger J, et al. Intracoronary stenting and angiographic results: strut thickness effect on restenosis outcome (ISAR-STEREO) trial. Circulation 2001;103:2816–21.

13. Pache J, Kastrati A, Mehilli J, et al. Intracoronary stenting and angiographic results: strut thickness effect on restenosis outcome (ISAR-STEREO-2) trial. J Am Coll Cardiol 2003;41:1283–8.

14. Gogas BD, McDaniel M, Samady H, et al. Novel drug-eluting stents for coronary revascularization. Trends Cardiovasc Med 2014;24:305–13.

15. Takebayashi H, Mintz GS, Carlier SG, et al. Nonuniform strut distribution correlates with more neointimal hyperplasia after sirolimus-eluting stent implantation. Circulation 2004;110:3430–4.

16. Kolandaivelu K, Leiden BB, Edelman ER. Predicting response to endovascular therapies: dissecting the roles of local lesion complexity, systemic comorbidity, and clinical uncertainty. J Biomech 2014;47:908–21.

17. Kolandaivelu K, Swaminathan R, Gibson WJ, et al. Stent thrombogenicity early in high-risk interventional settings is driven by stent design and deployment and protected by polymer-drug coatings. Circulation 2011;123:1400–9.

18. Joner M, Finn AV, Farb A, et al. Pathology of drug-eluting stents in humans: delayed healing and late thrombotic risk. J Am Coll Cardiol 2006;48:193–202.

19. Nebeker JR, Virmani R, Bennett CL, et al. Hypersensitivity cases associated with drug-eluting coronary stents: a review of available cases from the Research on Adverse Drug Events and Reports (RADAR) project. J Am Coll Cardiol 2006;47:175–81.

20. Kereiakes DJ, Meredith IT, Windecker S, et al. Efficacy and safety of a novel bioabsorbable polymer-coated, everolimus-eluting coronary stent: the EVOLVE II Randomized Trial. Circ Cardiovasc Interv 2015;8.

21. Huang Y, Ng HC, Ng XW, et al. Drug-eluting biostable and erodible stents. J Control Release 2014;193:188–201.

22. Finn AV, Nakazawa G, Joner M, et al. Vascular responses to drug eluting stents: importance of delayed healing. Arterioscler Thromb Vasc Biol 2007;27:1500–10.

23. Iqbal J, Gunn J, Serruys PW. Coronary stents: historical development, current status and future directions. Br Med Bull 2013;106:193–211.

24. Garg S, Serruys PW. Coronary stents: current status. J Am Coll Cardiol 2010;56:S1–42.

25. Stefanini GG, Taniwaki M, Windecker S. Coronary stents: novel developments. Heart 2014;100:1051–61.

26. Allocco DJ, Jacoski MV, Huibregtse B, et al. Platinum Chromium Stent Series â The TAXUS Element (ION), PROMUS Element and OMEGA Stents. Intervent Cardiol 2011;6:134–41.

27. Chhatriwalla AK, Cam A, Unzek S, et al. Drug-eluting stent fracture and acute coronary syndrome. Cardiovasc Revasc Med 2009;10:166–71.

28. Park KW, Park JJ, Chae IH, et al. Clinical characteristics of coronary drug-eluting stent fracture: insights from a two-center des registry. J Korean Med Sci 2011;26:53–8.

29. Mamas MA, Foin N, Abunassar C, et al. Stent fracture: Insights on mechanisms, treatments, and outcomes from the food and drug administration manufacturer and user facility device experience database. Catheter Cardiovasc Interv 2014;83:E251–9.

30. Nakazawa G, Finn AV, Vorpahl M, et al. Incidence and predictors of drug-eluting stent fracture in human coronary artery a pathologic analysis. J Am Coll Cardiol 2009;54:1924–31.

31. Chakravarty T, White AJ, Buch M, et al. Meta-analysis of incidence, clinical characteristics and implications of stent fracture. Am J Cardiol 2010;106:1075–80.

32. Everett KD, Conway C, Desany GJ, et al. Structural Mechanics Predictions Relating to Clinical Coronary Stent Fracture in a 5 Year Period in FDA MAUDE Database. Ann Biomed Eng 2016;44(2):391–403.

33. Park MW, Chang K, Her SH, et al. Incidence and clinical impact of fracture of drug-eluting stents widely used in current clinical practice: comparison with initial platform of sirolimus-eluting stent. J Cardiol 2012;60:215–21.

34. Mamas MA, Williams PD. Longitudinal stent deformation: insights on mechanisms, treatments and outcomes from the Food and Drug Administration Manufacturer and User Facility Device Experience database. EuroIntervention 2012;8:196–204.

35. Williams PD, Mamas MA, Morgan KP, et al. Longitudinal stent deformation: a retrospective analysis of frequency and mechanisms. EuroIntervention 2012;8:267–74.

36. Prabhu S, Schikorr T, Mahmoud T, et al. Engineering assessment of the longitudinal compression behaviour of contemporary coronary stents. EuroIntervention 2012;8:275–81.

37. Kereiakes DJ, Popma JJ, Cannon LA, et al. Longitudinal stent deformation: quantitative coronary angiographic analysis from the PERSEUS and PLATINUM randomised controlled clinical trials. EuroIntervention 2012;8:187–95.

38. Otsuka F, Vorpahl M, Nakano M, et al. Pathology of second-generation everolimus-eluting stents versus first-generation sirolimus- and paclitaxel-eluting stents in humans. Circulation 2014;129:211–23.

39. Iakovou I, Schmidt T, Bonizzoni E, et al. Incidence, predictors, and outcome of thrombosis after successful implantation of drug-eluting stents. JAMA 2005;293:2126–30.

40. van Werkum JW, Heestermans AA, de Korte FI, et al. Long-term clinical outcome after a first angiographically confirmed coronary stent thrombosis: an analysis of 431 cases. Circulation 2009;119: 828–34.

41. Stettler C, Wandel S, Allemann S, et al. Outcomes associated with drug-eluting and bare-metal stents: a collaborative network meta-analysis. Lancet 2007;370:937–48.

42. Stone GW, Moses JW, Ellis SG, et al. Safety and efficacy of sirolimus- and paclitaxel-eluting coronary stents. N Engl J Med 2007;356:998–1008.

43. Nakazawa G, Finn AV, Joner M, et al. Delayed arterial healing and increased late stent thrombosis at culprit sites after drug-eluting stent placement for acute myocardial infarction patients: an autopsy study. Circulation 2008;118:1138–45.

44. Stone GW, Ellis SG, Colombo A, et al. Offsetting impact of thrombosis and restenosis on the occurrence of death and myocardial infarction after paclitaxel-eluting and bare metal stent implantation. Circulation 2007;115:2842–7.

45. Nakazawa G, Finn AV, Vorpahl M, et al. Coronary responses and differential mechanisms of late stent thrombosis attributed to first-generation sirolimus- and paclitaxel-eluting stents. J Am Coll Cardiol 2011;57:390–8.

46. Palmerini T, Benedetto U, Biondi-Zoccai G, et al. Long-Term Safety of Drug-Eluting and Bare-Metal Stents: Evidence From a Comprehensive Network Meta-Analysis. J Am Coll Cardiol 2015; 65:2496–507.

47. Sabate M, Brugaletta S, Cequier A, et al. Clinical outcomes in patients with ST-segment elevation myocardial infarction treated with everolimus-eluting stents versus bare-metal stents (EXAMINATION): 5-year results of a randomised trial. Lancet 2016;387(10016):357–66.

48. Sabate M, Cequier A, Iniguez A, et al. Everolimus-eluting stent versus bare-metal stent in ST-segment elevation myocardial infarction (EXAMINATION): 1 year results of a randomised controlled trial. Lancet 2012;380:1482–90.

49. Kereiakes DJ, Yeh RW, Massaro JM, et al. Stent Thrombosis in Drug-Eluting or Bare-Metal Stents in Patients Receiving Dual Antiplatelet Therapy. JACC Cardiovasc Interv 2015;8:1552–62.

50. Kereiakes DJ, Cannon LA, Dauber I, et al. Long-term follow-up of the platinum chromium TAXUS element (ION) stent: The PERSEUS Workhorse and Small Vessel Trial Five-Year Results. Catheter Cardiovasc Interv 2015;86:994–1001.

51. Applegate RJ, Yaqub M, Hermiller JB, et al. Long-term (three-year) safety and efficacy of everolimus-eluting stents compared to paclitaxel-eluting stents (from the SPIRIT III Trial). Am J Cardiol 2011;107: 833–40.

52. Stone GW, Midei M, Newman W, et al. Randomized comparison of everolimus-eluting and paclitaxel-eluting stents: two-year clinical follow-up from the Clinical Evaluation of the Xience V Everolimus Eluting Coronary Stent System in the Treatment of Patients with de novo Native Coronary Artery Lesions (SPIRIT) III trial. Circulation 2009;119:680–6.

53. Stone GW, Midei M, Newman W, et al. Comparison of an everolimus-eluting stent and a paclitaxel-eluting stent in patients with coronary artery disease: a randomized trial. JAMA 2008; 299:1903–13.

54. Gada H, Kirtane AJ, Newman W, et al. 5-year results of a randomized comparison of XIENCE V everolimus-eluting and TAXUS paclitaxel-eluting stents: final results from the SPIRIT III trial (clinical evaluation of the XIENCE V everolimus eluting coronary stent system in the treatment of patients with de novo native coronary artery lesions). JACC Cardiovasc Interv 2013;6:1263–6.

55. Stone GW, Rizvi A, Newman W, et al. Everolimus-eluting versus paclitaxel-eluting stents in coronary artery disease. N Engl J Med 2010;362:1663–74.

56. Dangas GD, Serruys PW, Kereiakes DJ, et al. Meta-analysis of everolimus-eluting versus paclitaxel-eluting stents in coronary artery disease: final 3-year results of the SPIRIT clinical trials program (Clinical Evaluation of the Xience V Everolimus Eluting Coronary Stent System in the Treatment of Patients With De Novo Native Coronary Artery Lesions). JACC Cardiovasc Interv 2013;6:914–22.

57. Kaul U, Bangalore S, Seth A, et al. Paclitaxel-Eluting versus Everolimus-Eluting Coronary Stents in Diabetes. N Engl J Med 2015;373:1709–19.

58. Leon MB, Mauri L, Popma JJ, et al. A randomized comparison of the Endeavor zotarolimus-eluting stent versus the TAXUS paclitaxel-eluting stent in de novo native coronary lesions 12-month outcomes from the ENDEAVOR IV trial. J Am Coll Cardiol 2010;55:543–54.

59. Kirtane AJ, Leon MB, Ball MW, et al. The "final" 5-year follow-up from the ENDEAVOR IV trial comparing a zotarolimus-eluting stent with a paclitaxel-eluting stent. JACC Cardiovasc Interv 2013;6:325–33.

60. Kandzari DE, Mauri L, Popma JJ, et al. Late-term clinical outcomes with zotarolimus- and sirolimus-eluting stents. 5-year follow-up of the ENDEAVOR III (A Randomized Controlled Trial of the Medtronic Endeavor Drug [ABT-578] Eluting Coronary Stent System Versus the Cypher Sirolimus-Eluting Coronary Stent System in De Novo Native Coronary Artery Lesions). JACC Cardiovasc Interv 2011;4:543–50.

61. Maeng M, Tilsted HH, Jensen LO, et al. 3-Year clinical outcomes in the randomized SORT OUT III superiority trial comparing zotarolimus- and

sirolimus-eluting coronary stents. JACC Cardio-vasc Interv 2012;5:812–8.

62. Byrne RA, Kastrati A, Tiroch K, et al. 2-year clinical and angiographic outcomes from a randomized trial of polymer-free dual drug-eluting stents versus polymer-based Cypher and Endeavor [corrected] drug-eluting stents. J Am Coll Cardiol 2010;55: 2536–43.

63. Park DW, Kim YH, Yun SC, et al. Comparison of zotarolimus-eluting stents with sirolimus- and paclitaxel-eluting stents for coronary revascularization: the ZEST (comparison of the efficacy and safety of zotarolimus-eluting stent with sirolimus-eluting and paclitaxel-eluting stent for coronary lesions) randomized trial. J Am Coll Cardiol 2010;56: 1187–95.

64. Mauri L, Massaro JM, Jiang S, et al. Long-term clinical outcomes with zotarolimus-eluting versus bare-metal coronary stents. JACC Cardiovasc Interv 2010;3:1240–9.

65. Kandzari DE, Leon MB, Meredith I, et al. Final 5-year outcomes from the Endeavor zotarolimus-eluting stent clinical trial program: comparison of safety and efficacy with first-generation drug-eluting and bare-metal stents. JACC Cardiovasc Interv 2013;6:504–12.

66. Maeng M, Tilsted HH, Jensen LO, et al. Differential clinical outcomes after 1 year versus 5 years in a randomised comparison of zotarolimus-eluting and sirolimus-eluting coronary stents (the SORT OUT III study): a multicentre, open-label, randomised superiority trial. Lancet 2014;383: 2047–56.

67. Wijns W, Steg PG, Mauri L, et al. Endeavour zotarolimus-eluting stent reduces stent thrombosis and improves clinical outcomes compared with cypher sirolimus-eluting stent: 4-year results of the PROTECT randomized trial. Eur Heart J 2014; 35:2812–20.

68. Meredith IT, Worthley S, Whitbourn R, et al. Clinical and angiographic results with the next-generation resolute stent system: a prospective, multicenter, first-in-human trial. JACC Cardiovasc Interv 2009; 2:977–85.

69. Meredith IT, Worthley SG, Whitbourn R, et al. Long-term clinical outcomes with the next-generation Resolute Stent System: a report of the two-year follow-up from the RESOLUTE clinical trial. EuroIntervention 2010;5:692–7.

70. Serruys PW, Silber S, Garg S, et al. Comparison of zotarolimus-eluting and everolimus-eluting coronary stents. N Engl J Med 2010;363:136–46.

71. Iqbal J, Serruys PW, Silber S, et al. Comparison of zotarolimus- and everolimus-eluting coronary stents: final 5-year report of the RESOLUTE all-comers trial. Circ Cardiovasc Interv 2015;8: e002230.

72. von Birgelen C, Basalus MW, Tandjung K, et al. A randomized controlled trial in second-generation zotarolimus-eluting Resolute stents versus everolimus-eluting Xience V stents in real-world patients: the TWENTE trial. J Am Coll Cardiol 2012;59:1350–61.

73. Tsuchida K, Piek JJ, Neumann FJ, et al. One-year results of a durable polymer everolimus-eluting stent in de novo coronary narrowings (The SPIRIT FIRST Trial). EuroIntervention 2005;1:266–72.

74. Bangalore S, Kumar S, Fusaro M, et al. Short- and long-term outcomes with drug-eluting and bare-metal coronary stents: a mixed-treatment comparison analysis of 117 762 patient-years of follow-up from randomized trials. Circulation 2012;125: 2873–91.

75. Palmerini T, Biondi-Zoccai G, Della Riva D, et al. Stent thrombosis with drug-eluting and bare-metal stents: evidence from a comprehensive network meta-analysis. Lancet 2012;379:1393–402.

76. Smits PC, Vlachojannis GJ, McFadden EP, et al. Final 5-Year Follow-Up of a Randomized Controlled Trial of Everolimus- and Paclitaxel-Eluting Stents for Coronary Revascularization in Daily Practice: The COMPARE Trial (A Trial of Everolimus-Eluting Stents and Paclitaxel Stents for Coronary Revascularization in Daily Practice). JACC Cardiovasc Interv 2015;8:1157–65.

77. Kimura T, Morimoto T, Natsuaki M, et al. Comparison of everolimus-eluting and sirolimus-eluting coronary stents: 1-year outcomes from the Randomized Evaluation of Sirolimus-eluting Versus Everolimus-eluting stent Trial (RESET). Circulation 2012;126:1225–36.

78. Kaiser C, Galatius S, Erne P, et al. Drug-eluting versus bare-metal stents in large coronary arteries. N Engl J Med 2010;363:2310–9.

79. Park KW, Chae IH, Lim DS, et al. Everolimus-eluting versus sirolimus-eluting stents in patients undergoing percutaneous coronary intervention: the EXCELLENT (Efficacy of Xience/Promus Versus Cypher to Reduce Late Loss After Stenting) randomized trial. J Am Coll Cardiol 2011;58:1844–54.

80. Jensen LO, Thayssen P, Maeng M, et al. Three-year outcomes after revascularization with everolimus- and sirolimus-eluting stents from the SORT OUT IV trial. JACC Cardiovasc Interv 2014;7:840–8.

81. Baber U, Mehran R, Sharma SK, et al. Impact of the everolimus-eluting stent on stent thrombosis: a meta-analysis of 13 randomized trials. J Am Coll Cardiol 2011;58:1569–77.

82. Stone GW, Teirstein PS, Meredith IT, et al. A prospective, randomized evaluation of a novel everolimus-eluting coronary stent: the PLATINUM (a Prospective, Randomized, Multicenter Trial to Assess an Everolimus-Eluting Coronary Stent System [PROMUS Element] for the Treatment of Up

to Two de Novo Coronary Artery Lesions) trial. J Am Coll Cardiol 2011;57:1700–8.

83. Meredith IT, Teirstein PS, Bouchard A, et al. Three-year results comparing platinum-chromium PRO-MUS element and cobalt-chromium XIENCE V everolimus-eluting stents in de novo coronary artery narrowing (from the PLATINUM Trial). Am J Cardiol 2014;113:1117–23.

84. von Birgelen C, Sen H, Lam MK, et al. Third-generation zotarolimus-eluting and everolimus-eluting stents in all-comer patients requiring a percutaneous coronary intervention (DUTCH PEERS): a randomised, single-blind, multicentre, non-inferiority trial. Lancet 2014;383:413–23.

85. Park KW, Kang SH, Kang HJ, et al. A randomized comparison of platinum chromium-based everolimus-eluting stents versus cobalt chromium-based Zotarolimus-Eluting stents in all-comers receiving percutaneous coronary intervention: HOST-ASSURE (harmonizing optimal strategy for treatment of coronary artery stenosis-safety & effectiveness of drug-eluting stents & antiplatelet regimen), a randomized, controlled, non-inferiority trial. J Am Coll Cardiol 2014;63:2805–16.

86. Kalesan B, Pilgrim T, Heinimann K, et al. Comparison of drug-eluting stents with bare metal stents in patients with ST-segment elevation myocardial infarction. Eur Heart J 2012;33:977–87.

87. Guo N, Maehara A, Mintz GS, et al. Incidence, mechanisms, predictors, and clinical impact of acute and late stent malapposition after primary intervention in patients with acute myocardial infarction: an intravascular ultrasound substudy of the Harmonizing Outcomes with Revascularization and Stents in Acute Myocardial Infarction (HORIZONS-AMI) trial. Circulation 2010;122:1077–84.

88. Hwang CW, Levin AD, Jonas M, et al. Thrombosis modulates arterial drug distribution for drug-eluting stents. Circulation 2005;111:1619–26.

89. Balakrishnan B, Dooley J, Kopia G, et al. Thrombus causes fluctuations in arterial drug delivery from intravascular stents. J Control Release 2008;131:173–80.

90. Di Lorenzo E, Sauro R, Varricchio A, et al. Randomized comparison of everolimus-eluting stents and sirolimus-eluting stents in patients with ST elevation myocardial infarction: RACES-MI trial. JACC Cardiovasc Interv 2014;7:849–56.

91. Hofma SH, Brouwer J, Velders MA, et al. Second-generation everolimus-eluting stents versus first-generation sirolimus-eluting stents in acute myocardial infarction. 1-year results of the randomized XAMI (XienceV Stent vs. Cypher Stent in Primary PCI for Acute Myocardial Infarction) trial. J Am Coll Cardiol 2012;60:381–7.

92. Palmerini T, Biondi-Zoccai G, Della Riva D, et al. Clinical outcomes with drug-eluting and bare-metal stents in patients with ST-segment elevation myocardial infarction: evidence from a comprehensive network meta-analysis. J Am Coll Cardiol 2013;62:496–504.

93. Wang L, Zang W, Xie D, et al. Drug-eluting stents for acute coronary syndrome: a meta-analysis of randomized controlled trials. PLoS One 2013;8:e72895.

94. Green SM, Selzer F, Mulukutla SR, et al. Comparison of bare-metal and drug-eluting stents in patients with chronic kidney disease (from the NHLBI Dynamic Registry). Am J Cardiol 2011;108:1658–64.

95. Kahn MR, Robbins MJ, Kim MC, et al. Management of cardiovascular disease in patients with kidney disease. Nat Rev Cardiol 2013;10:261–73.

96. Simsek C, Magro M, Boersma E, et al. Impact of renal insufficiency on safety and efficacy of drug-eluting stents compared to bare-metal stents at 6 years. Catheter Cardiovasc Interv 2012;80:18–26.

97. Tsai TT, Messenger JC, Brennan JM, et al. Safety and efficacy of drug-eluting stents in older patients with chronic kidney disease: a report from the linked CathPCI Registry-CMS claims database. J Am Coll Cardiol 2011;58:1859–69.

98. Stettler C, Allemann S, Wandel S, et al. Drug eluting and bare metal stents in people with and without diabetes: collaborative network meta-analysis. BMJ 2008;337:a1331.

99. Bangalore S, Kumar S, Fusaro M, et al. Outcomes with various drug eluting or bare metal stents in patients with diabetes mellitus: mixed treatment comparison analysis of 22,844 patient years of follow-up from randomised trials. BMJ 2012;345:e5170.

100. Vardi M, Burke DA, Bangalore S, et al. Long-term efficacy and safety of Zotarolimus-eluting stent in patients with diabetes mellitus: pooled 5-year results from the ENDEAVOR III and IV trials. Catheter Cardiovasc Interv 2013;82:1031–8.

Left Atrial Appendage Closure Device in Atrial Fibrillation

Michael C. Giudici, MD, FHRS*, Prashant D. Bhave, MD, FHRS

KEYWORDS

- Left atrial appendage closure • Anticoagulation • Embolic stroke

KEY POINTS

- Left atrial appendage closure is an attractive, but unproven technology.
- Warfarin has a 50-year track record of success in prevention of embolic stroke.
- If it ain't broke, don't fix it.

There are known knowns. These are things we know that we know. There are known unknowns. That is to say, there are things that we know we don't know. But there are also unknown unknowns. These are things we don't know we don't know.

—Donald Rumsfeld

Case History

A 76 y/o patient has been on anticoagulation with warfarin for thromboembolic prophylaxis for atrial fibrillation for the past 3 years and has had no complications. The CHADS2 score is 3 for HTN and DM and age. There has not been a thromboembolic event and no bleeding complications. The INR measurements, however, have fluctuated over the years. You recommend placement of a WATCHMAN left atrial appendage closure device and discontinuation of warfarin.

I have been asked to make a case against implanting a Watchman device (Boston Scientific Corporation, Natick, MA) at this time in this asymptomatic 76-year-old man who seems to be getting along well on warfarin, albeit with some lability in international normalized ratio (INR) values.

When we as physicians consider any therapy for a patient, we evaluate the therapy on the basis of its safety, its efficacy, and its cost.

SAFETY

Let's start with the known knowns. Warfarin has been used as an oral anticoagulant for more than half a century. If you try to list medications that have been widely used as long as warfarin, only penicillin and aspirin come to mind. The number of patients treated with warfarin over the years would be in the millions. To list all the trials over the years in which investigators tried to find something as safe and efficacious as warfarin is beyond the scope of this article. The Stroke Prevention in Atrial Fibrillation Trials (SPAF)[1] and the ACTIVE trials[2] were among the largest that failed to bump warfarin off the top step of the podium. It was not until the new "novel" anticoagulants came along that we have a therapy that is potentially as safe and effective as warfarin.[3–5] Warfarin is an easy drug to dislike. The issues with drug and diet interactions,

---

This article originally appeared in Cardiac Electrophysiology Clinics, Volume 7, Issue 3, September 2015.

The authors have no conflicts of interest to disclose.

Division of Cardiovascular Medicine, Department of Internal Medicine, University of Iowa Hospitals and Clinics, 200 Hawkins Drive, Iowa City, IA 52242, USA

* Corresponding author. 200 Hawkins Drive, 4426JCP, Iowa City, IA 52242.

E-mail address: michael-c-giudici@uiowa.edu

the need for constant monitoring, and its relatively narrow therapeutic range drive the search for potential alternatives.[6,7] And there is still a residual risk of stroke despite optimal anticoagulation.[8]

That is not to say that there are no safety issues. In SPAF, there was a 1.2% per year risk of "relevant hemorrhage" on warfarin. That was not significantly different from aspirin or placebo, however. In the PROTECT-AF WATCHMAN Trial[9] there was 7.4% risk of major bleeding in the warfarin group over 2612 patient-years (45 months) of follow-up.

We know that warfarin is well-tolerated compared with other medications. It very rarely will cause a rash or gastrointestinal upset. We also know that INRs may fluctuate in a number of patients and that is associated with its own risks. In the SPAF III trial,[10] 7 of 12 major bleeds occurred in patients with INRs greater than 3.0. Likewise, if the INR is low, the risk of stroke increases. Hylek[11] demonstrated a 3.3 times greater risk of stroke if the INR was 1.5 compared with 2.0.

What do we know about the safety of the Watchman device? In the PROTECT-AF Trial, the procedural success was only 91%. This means that 9% of patients were exposed to the risk of a procedure and did not receive the device. In addition, 4.8% had "serious pericardial effusion," 1.3% had procedural stroke, and 0.6% had device embolization. Over the course of the 45-month follow-up, 4.8% had major bleeding and 0.6% had hemorrhagic stroke compared with 7.4% and 3.7%, respectively, on warfarin. We also know that as physicians gained experience with placement of the device, the procedural complication rates decreased. In the continued access arm of the PROTECT-AF Trial (CAP),[12] the rate of procedure-related or device-related safety events within the first 7 days of the procedure decreased to 3.7% from 7.7% in the initial trial. The rate of serious pericardial effusion within 7 days of the procedure decreased to 2.2% from 5.0%.

What are the known unknowns? These would mainly be with regard to long-term safety and efficacy of the Watchman device. What is the risk of device erosion through the wall of the atrium? What is the risk that leaks into the appendage will develop over time? There are reports[13,14] suggesting that progressive increases in peridevice leakage are associated with an increase in the incidence of stroke. There also are reports of the device itself being a source of thrombus. Will future modifications to the device eliminate that problem?

And as long as we are comparing pharmacologic therapy with device therapy, what would be the long-term comparison of the non–vitamin K antagonist anticoagulant agents with an appendage-occluding device in this patient with fluctuating INRs?

The unknown unknowns? We just don't know....

EFFICACY

The known knowns.... In SPAF, the primary events were ischemic stroke and systemic embolism. During a mean follow-up of 1.3 years, a relatively short time frame, the rate of primary events in patients assigned to placebo was 7.4% versus 2.3% in the warfarin group. In the ACTIVE-W Trial, compared with warfarin therapy, use of clopidogrel/aspirin was associated with a 45% increase in the risk of the primary endpoints of stroke, non-central nervous system (CNS) embolism, myocardial infarction, and vascular death (annual rates for events, 3.93% vs 5.64%, respectively; $P = .0002$). This difference was driven by significantly higher incidences of stroke and non-CNS embolism in the clopidogrel/aspirin arm. The cumulative risk of major bleeding complications was nearly identical in the clopidogrel/aspirin and warfarin groups (2.4% vs 2.2% per year, respectively; $P = .67$).

The Watchman device has been likewise shown to be reasonably effective in prevention of stroke. In the PROTECT-AF Trial, the primary endpoints were stroke, systemic embolization, and cardiovascular (CV) death. Set up as a noninferiority trial, in 1.8 years of follow-up the primary endpoint was met in 3.0% of patients randomized to the Watchman device and 4.9% in the warfarin group (Relative Risk (RR) 0.62). With longer follow-up to 45 months, the primary endpoint was met with 2.3 events per 100 patient-years in the Watchman group and 3.8 events per 100 patient-years for patients randomized to warfarin (RR 0.6).

In the PREVAIL trial, which also compared the Watchman device with warfarin therapy, the procedural success rate had increased to 95.1% with more experience with the device. However, the primary endpoints of stroke, systemic embolism, and CV and unexplained death did not meet noninferiority criteria (RR 1.07) at 18-month follow-up, although there was not a great difference in outcomes between the 2 groups.[15]

The known unknowns would be the same as those mentioned previously. We do not have long-term follow-up of the Watchman device. What are the late complications? What is the long-term efficacy? Is occluding the ostium of a functioning left appendage a good thing to do, or should we just remove it? Where else do clots form?

COSTS

There are some data regarding costs of these therapies.[16] Because both left atrial appendage closure devices and the novel oral anticoagulants are relatively new, cost analysis is done in present-day dollars and modeling is used. A study done by Boston Scientific in Europe suggested that the Watchman device was 10% more expensive than warfarin over a 10-year period.[17] When comparing warfarin with the novel oral anticoagulants, warfarin was still most cost-effective, although one analysis determined that the novel agents produced a greater quality-adjusted life expectancy than warfarin.[18]

Are there unknown late costs to left atrial appendage (LAA) occlusion device therapy? We do not have data on 10-year-old Watchman implants. We do have data on patients on warfarin for 10 years.

DISCUSSION

So what do we do with our asymptomatic patient? In general, we do not do procedures with significant risk on asymptomatic patients unless they have a potentially life-threatening problem, such as a rapidly conducting accessory pathway (catheter ablation) or significant risk of sudden cardiac arrest (implantable cardioverter defibrillator [ICD] placement). One could argue that accessory pathway ablation and ICD placement also carry less procedural risk at this time than LAA closure device placement.

If the concern with this patient is his fluctuating INRs, why not just change to a novel anticoagulant? Problem solved without a procedure….

If a procedure is felt to be indicated, then is Watchman placement the best option? A recent report by Mora and colleagues[19] demonstrated that 7 months after a successful Lariat (Sentre-HEART, Inc, Redwood City, CA) procedure, the appendage was essentially gone. This would mean there is no risk of progressive leakage around the device or risk of erosion. To be fair, however, the Lariat device also has been associated with incomplete occlusion and leakage in up to 20%, and presence of thrombus in 4.8%.[20]

And what about the unknown unknowns? Are we treating the right thing by doing LAA closure? Will this go down in history like the internal mammary artery ligation procedure[21] (a surgery done in the 1950s in which the internal mammary artery was ligated to "increase coronary blood flow and relieve angina pectoris") after we find that people still have strokes from another source? What else is out there for us to learn about the relationship

of atrial fibrillation (AF) and stroke? The ASSERT and TRENDS trials[22,23] seem to open Pandora's Box. In both of these studies of patients with cardiac devices (pacemakers or ICDs) and newly diagnosed atrial tachyarrhythmia/AF, there was a very poor temporal relationship between atrial arrhythmia episodes and timing of embolic events.

SUMMARY

We have come a long way but still seem to have a long way to go in completely understanding the relationship between AF and stroke. I would suggest that if this gentleman is happy with his current therapy, he should stay on his current therapy.

REFERENCES

1. Stroke Prevention in Atrial Fibrillation Investigators. Stroke prevention in atrial fibrillation study. Final results. Circulation 1991;84(2):527–39.
2. The ACTIVE Writing Group on behalf of the ACTIVE Investigators. Clopidogrel plus aspirin versus oral anticoagulation for atrial fibrillation in the atrial fibrillation clopidogrel trial with Irbesartan for prevention of vascular events (ACTIVE W): a randomised controlled trial. Lancet 2006; 367(9526):1903–12.
3. Connolly SJ, Ezekowitz MD, Yusuf S, et al. Dabigatran versus warfarin in patients with atrial fibrillation. N Engl J Med 2009;361(12):1139–51.
4. Flaker G, Lopes RD, Hylek E, et al. Amiodarone, anticoagulation, and clinical events in patients with atrial fibrillation: insights from the ARISTOTLE trial. J Am Coll Cardiol 2014;64(15):1541–50.
5. Patel MR, Mahaffey KW, Garg J, et al. Rivaroxaban versus warfarin in nonvalvular atrial fibrillation. N Engl J Med 2011;365(10):883–91.
6. Holbrook AM, Pereira JA, Labiris R, et al. Systematic overview of warfarin and its drug and food interactions. Arch Intern Med 2005;165(10):1095–106.
7. Gersh BJ, Freedman JE, Granger CB. Antiplatelet and anticoagulant therapy for stroke prevention in patients with non-valvular atrial fibrillation: evidence based strategies and new developments. Rev Esp Cardiol 2011;64(4):260–8 [in Spanish].
8. Ahrens I, Lip GY, Peter K. What do the RE-LY, AVERROES and ROCKET-AF trials tell us for stroke prevention in atrial fibrillation? Thromb Haemost 2011; 105(4):574–8.
9. Reddy VY, Sievert H, Halperin J, et al. Percutaneous left atrial appendage closure vs warfarin for atrial fibrillation: a randomized clinical trial. JAMA 2014; 312(19):1988–98.
10. Patients with nonvalvular atrial fibrillation at low risk of stroke during treatment with aspirin: Stroke prevention in atrial fibrillation III study. The SPAF III writing

committee for the stroke prevention in atrial fibrillation investigators. JAMA 1998;279(16):1273–7.

11. Hylek EM. Vitamin K antagonists and time in the therapeutic range: implications, challenges, and strategies for improvement. J Thromb Thrombolysis 2013;35(3):333–5.

12. Reddy VY, Holmes D, Doshi SK, et al. Safety of percutaneous left atrial appendage closure: results from the Watchman Left Atrial Appendage System for Embolic Protection in Patients with AF (PROTECT AF) clinical trial and the Continued Access Registry. Circulation 2011;123(4):417–24.

13. Lee K, Park SJ, Kwon HJ, et al. Progressive increase in peridevice leakage after the implantation of the watchman device on long-term serial echocardiographic follow-up. Can J Cardiol 2014;30(11):1461. e15–7.

14. Viles-Gonzalez JF, Kar S, Douglas P, et al. The clinical impact of incomplete left atrial appendage closure with the Watchman device in patients with atrial fibrillation: a PROTECT AF (Percutaneous Closure of the Left Atrial Appendage versus Warfarin Therapy for Prevention of Stroke in Patients with Atrial Fibrillation) substudy. J Am Coll Cardiol 2012; 59(10):923–9.

15. Holmes DR Jr, Kar S, Price MJ, et al. Prospective randomized evaluation of the Watchman Left Atrial Appendage Closure device in patients with atrial fibrillation versus long-term warfarin therapy: the PREVAIL trial. J Am Coll Cardiol 2014;64(1):1–12.

16. Coyle D, Coyle K, Cameron C, et al. Cost-effectiveness of new oral anticoagulants compared with warfarin in preventing stroke and other cardiovascular events in patients with atrial fibrillation. Value Health 2013;16(4):498–506.

17. Amorosi SL, Armstrong S, Da Deppo L, et al. The budget impact of left atrial appendage closure compared with adjusted-dose warfarin and dabigatran etexilate for stroke prevention in atrial fibrillation. Europace 2014;16(8):1131–6.

18. Canestaro WJ, Patrick AR, Avorn J, et al. Cost-effectiveness of oral anticoagulants for treatment of atrial fibrillation. Circ Cardiovasc Qual Outcomes 2013; 6(6):724–31.

19. Mora L, Merchant FM, Delurgio DB, et al. First gross anatomical description in human of left atrial appendage involution after LARIAT procedure. J Cardiovasc Electrophysiol 2014;26(3):350–1.

20. Price MJ, Gibson DN, Yakubov SJ, et al. Early safety and efficacy of percutaneous left atrial appendage suture ligation: results from the US transcatheter LAA ligation consortium. J Am Coll Cardiol 2014; 64(6):565–72.

21. Glover RP, Davila JC, Kyle RH, et al. Ligation of the internal mammary arteries as a means of increasing blood supply to the myocardium. J Thorac Surg 1957;34(5):661–78.

22. Brambatti M, Connolly SJ, Gold MR, et al. Temporal relationship between subclinical atrial fibrillation and embolic events. Circulation 2014;129(21):2094–9.

23. Daoud EG, Glotzer TV, Wyse DG, et al. Temporal relationship of atrial tachyarrhythmias, cerebrovascular events, and systemic emboli based on stored device data: a subgroup analysis of TRENDS. Heart Rhythm 2011;8(9):1416–23.

Index

Note: Page numbers of article titles are in **boldface** type.

cardiology.theclinics.com

Moving?

Make sure your subscription moves with you!

To notify us of your new address, find your **Clinics Account Number** (located on your mailing label above your name), and contact customer service at:

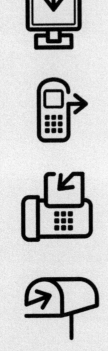

Email: journalscustomerservice-usa@elsevier.com

800-654-2452 (subscribers in the U.S. & Canada)
314-447-8871 (subscribers outside of the U.S. & Canada)

Fax number: 314-447-8029

Elsevier Health Sciences Division
Subscription Customer Service
3251 Riverport Lane
Maryland Heights, MO 63043

ELSEVIER

Printed and bound by CPI Group (UK) Ltd, Croydon, CR0 4YY

03/10/2024

01040302-0008